Ophthalmic Nursing Standards & Procedures

Lynn Ring
Miriam Okoro

Ophthalmic Nursing Standards & Procedures
Lynn Ring and Miriam Okoro

ISBN: 978-1-905539-79-6

First published 2012

British Library Cataloguing in Publication Data
A catalogue record for this book is available from the British Library

Notice

Clinical practice and medical knowledge constantly evolve. Standard safety precautions must be followed, but, as knowledge is broadened by research, changes in practice, treatment and drug therapy may become necessary or appropriate. Readers must check the most current product information provided by the manufacturer of each drug to be administered and verify the dosages and correct administration, as well as contraindications. It is the responsibility of the practitioner, utilising the experience and knowledge of the patient, to determine dosages and the best treatment for each individual patient. Any brands mentioned in this book are as examples only and are not endorsed by the publisher. Neither the publisher nor the authors assume any liability for any injury and/or damage to persons or property arising from this publication.

To contact M&K Publishing write to:
M&K Update Ltd · The Old Bakery · St. John's Street
Keswick · Cumbria CA12 5AS
Tel: 01768 773030 · Fax: 01768 781099
publishing@mkupdate.co.uk
www.mkupdate.co.uk

Designed and typeset by Mary Blood
Printed in England by Ferguson Print, Keswick

Ophthalmic Nursing Standards & Procedures

Other books from M&K include:

Eye Emergencies: The practitioner's guide

ISBN: 978-1-905539-08-6

The Ophthalmic Study Guide

ISBN: 978-1-905539-40-6

Issues in Ophthalmic Practice: Current and future challenges

ISBN: 978-1-905539-17-8

Preoperative Assessment & Perioperative Management

ISBN: 978-1-905539-02-4

Nurses and Their Patients: Informing practice through psychodynamic insights

ISBN: 978-1-905539-31-4

Research Issues in Health and Social Care

ISBN: 978-1-905539-20-8

Preventing and Reducing Aggression & Violence in Health and Social Care: A holistic approach

ISBN: 978-1-905539-57-4

The ECG Workbook 2/e

ISBN: 978-1-905539-77-2

Contents

About the authors

Lynn Ring MSc, BSc (Hons), RN1, RNT, IP, ENB 346

Currently works at advanced level specialising in glaucoma, Accident & Emergency and developing diagnostic skills in diabetic retinopathy. She has been a member of the International Ophthalmic Nursing Association Council since 2010 and has articles published in the *International Journal of Ophthalmic Practice*.

Miriam Okoro MSc, Dip Management, RN1, SEN, ONC, 998, G&G 7300

Currently works as manager of an ophthalmic day case unit. She helps deliver an ophthalmic nursing course locally with an emphasis on competence in practice for registered nurses with a view to starting a non-registered ophthalmic nurse's course.

Introduction

This handbook of ophthalmic nursing procedures has been developed to assist the nurse/healthcare professional working in an ophthalmic environment and to provide the patient with safe and consistent ophthalmic nursing care. We discovered within our own unit that healthcare professionals, both registered and non-registered joining our workforce were often shown slightly different ways of doing things by the more experienced members of the team, leading to confusion for the new starter. We felt it was a bit like driving; bad habits can slip into everyday practice and although not unsafe, it was at times contradictory. So we went back to basics and developed standards of care which act as the benchmark for the ophthalmic practitioner.

At a recent conference, the back to basics call was reiterated by many of the delegates who confirmed that standards were slipping for a variety of reasons. Many identified the need for standards and we have developed this guide that provides the practitioner with a collection of written standards so that benchmarking can take place. Each standard was designed using the Royal College of Nursing Dynamic Standard Setting System (DySSSy) (RCN, 1990): Structure, Process, Outcome format. This system has been evaluated and found to improve quality of care through standard setting and audit of practice (Morrell *et al.* 1997).

However ophthalmic care is constantly changing and progressing with additional technical roles being introduced. There are some standards for using specific equipment detailed within this guide but we recommend that all practitioners become familiar with the manuals provided for specific equipment within their own workplace. We do not believe that this guide is exhaustive but should be used as an additional resource in conjunction with equipment manuals, other textbooks, local policies and guidelines.

We anticipate that these standards may help healthcare professionals (HCP) audit clinical practice whether as a registered nurse, healthcare assistant or ophthalmic technician and as such are available as guidance for benchmarking practice. The overall aim is to consistently meet the highest standard and be able to ensure ophthalmic care is evidence based as outlined by the principles of Clinical Governance (Department of Health, 1998).

All the guidance has been written using the term healthcare professional (HCP) which specifically relates to all staff working with ophthalmic patients regardless of registration. Non-registered practitioners are specifically highlighted in relation to prescription only medicines (POM) when we remind the reader to comply with local policy which may need a countersignature from a registered nurse or other such additional step even following satisfactory competence assessment. We hope that using clinical guidance like this helps the HCP to provide effective, efficient ophthalmic care.

We would like to remind the reader that informed consent is required for all procedures. Consent may take different forms for different procedures including written and verbal. Each procedure outlines in the first instance the need to obtain consent and the individual practitioner must ensure sufficient information is discussed to ensure the patient agrees to the procedure and consents to it taking place. In many instances this will take the form of verbal consent but if written consent is required, the reader is reminded to ensure adherence to local policy.

Many thanks are extended to all our colleagues who have supported us in the development of this set of standards. Particular thanks to Mr R. Wade, photographer and Mrs F. Selby, our willing volunteer who helped us with all the photos contained within the guide and to Prof. D. Field who became our unofficial reader to ensure we remained on the right track.

We hope you find this book both interesting and informative, using it to assist with benchmarking practice across the specialty. We have added an example of how we have competency assured the staff working within our units to encourage you to reflect on clinical practice.

Declaration: The authors have no commercial interest in any of the products outlined within this book. The authors intend to outline the standards for the particular equipment available within their workplace and recommend all readers to refer to the handbooks or manuals available within their own workplace for the specific equipment that they use.

Communication

Communication is a wide and varied subject that we do not intend to discuss in depth within this handbook. We intend to discuss communication from the perspective of the ophthalmic nurse using a common sense approach that has guided our practice for many years working within the ophthalmic arena.

Ophthalmology as a specialty includes a wide range of patients from all age groups and walks of life, with differing levels of visual ability, from acute A&E attendances to long-term chronic follow up. However they all have one thing in common – an eye problem which can cause extremes of anxiety and distress for conditions which we sometimes view as 'minor'.

In our experience, most people will experience a level of anxiety relating to any eye disease and their ability to manage this stressor can be enhanced by using effective communication skills. It is important to help the patient become involved as we need to elicit accurate information from them. An example springs to mind about how a patient reacts within a stressful situation although admittedly not linked to ophthalmology.

> A very stressful situation caused a lady to hyperventilate, feel dizzy and unsteady. She was attended by an efficient and kind healthcare professional, making the lady comfortable before asking about her medical history. The lady proceeded to explain that she had angina and an enlarged heart. This was news to the relative accompanying the lady. It was half an hour later before the lady realised she had given a detailed medical history for her mother rather than herself…

Stress and anxiety create a variety of responses from each individual so it is up to us, as the ophthalmic nurse, to ensure we create an environment which allows our patient to relax and impart accurate information. This assists with clinical decision making, developing an effective professional–patient relationship and ultimately improving the patient experience.

Most books relating to ophthalmology will include some information about communicating with visually impaired people. Madge (2006a) suggests an introduction of oneself to the patient should be 'followed by a relevant preamble' before taking a history from the patient. It is uncertain what a relevant preamble is.

Many ophthalmic nursing books allow the nurse to explore appropriate strategies to enhance effective communication with visually impaired people. Shaw et al, (2010), identifies communication 'etiquette' suggesting that the HCP is within the patient's field of vision, using a quiet room, free from distraction, addressing the patient not the carer if accompanied and avoiding shouting as most patients have retained their other senses. The first step in the process is to introduce yourself, clearly identify your role and say that you will be asking some questions before seeing the doctor or other clinical specialist for the complete clinical examination.

However it is important to remember that many non-verbal communication clues may be missed by patients with significant visual impairment (Whitaker, 2006). It might be advisable to start with a small amount of 'small talk', perhaps about the weather to help relax the patient and show you are solely interested in them at that moment. The patient in front of you should be the most important aspect of your professional life at that point in time. Be aware that sometimes it is possible to appear to be talking to the medical records rather than the patient if there is an absence of eye contact and perceived interest from the patient's perspective. Accurate documentation is important but the ophthalmic nurse needs to create a sense of 'being there' for each patient by making eye contact, smiling encouragingly, leaning a little forwards as if you are interested, ensuring you do not invade someone's personal space. Offer your hand as a greeting as you introduce yourself but ensure you only use touch appropriately. Use a common sense approach to touch – some patients interpret touch as a comforting or relaxing gesture whilst others may find touch inappropriate. The patient is only interested in the quality of the time spent with you.

You will have to clarify some things using open questioning techniques to ensure you have accurate information; however there is little need to repeat everything the patient has said to you. Try to summarise the salient facts. In today's busy clinics it may be tempting to allow the patient uninterrupted time to wander through their entire life history but actually you only have a few minutes to determine the relevant details. You can interrupt a patient albeit with tact and return the patient to the point in question. One way to do this is to use a closed question or paraphrase the most recent point.

Every patient is different and will need a slightly different approach. If you use these tips to build a rapport with your patient combined with some common sense and good manners, you will most likely obtain the information you need and improve the patient experience. The National Patient Survey (Department of Health, 2008) which explores the patient experience within NHS institutions showed that patients have six main factors when choosing which hospital to attend:

- Hospital cleanliness and low infection rates (74%)
- Quality of care (64%)
- Waiting times (63%)
- Friendliness of staff (57%)
- Reputation (55%)
- Ease of transport links/location (54%)

These are important factors for the ophthalmic nurse as we usually provide the first impression of any unit and it is worth noting that 57% of patients included manners and courtesy (friendliness of staff) as an important factor in their choice. We are all responsible for the reputation of our unit and common sense dictates that simple good manners initiate a positive first impression.

A group of ophthalmic nurses undertook a survey across three different NHS Trusts which prioritised the qualities of a 'good' eye nurse from the patients' perspective. The results showed that patients want us to be knowledgeable, skilled and competent; an excellent communicator; someone who listens and pays attention; someone who is empathetic and gives sound advice; honest and trustworthy; warm and friendly (Ring, 2010). This may sound impossible to achieve in a busy clinic or day surgery unit but we should all be aspiring to deliver care from the patient's perspective, particularly when we need to be effective communicators during history taking and patient education.

History Taking

All authors identify the composition of a 'good' history (Shaw *et al.* 2010; Marsden, 2007; Ledford, 1999). It consists of:

- Presenting condition – why has the patient arrived or been referred to the eye casualty or outpatient clinic?

- Past ophthalmic history – is there anything that might be contributing to this episode of care?
- Past medical history – is there a element of other medical problems that is likely to impact or create ophthalmic problems?
- Medications – are there current medications that could cause ophthalmic problems or impact on future prescribing?
- Allergies – this will influence a prescriber's choice of treatment.
- Family ophthalmic history – do any members of the family have ophthalmic problems with a familial or genetic component?
- Occupation – could the ophthalmic condition have an impact on employment or is the occupation impacting on the condition?
- Hobbies – has the ophthalmic condition impacted on any hobbies such as reading or sewing?
- Driving status – this may impede the ability of the ophthalmic nurse to dilate the pupils appropriately or the nurse may need to assess the visual acuity and how it relates to the current DVLA driving standards.
- Other social history – include smoking, alcohol consumption, recreational drug use as they all may impact on visual function; identify the patient who lives alone and may need additional support.

This list is not exhaustive. You may need to ask additional questions within your own workplace and you should always act in accordance with any specific local guidance and policy. All these details will, however, assist the doctor or HCP with clinical decision making as you will have clearly documented this in the individual's medical records (NMC, 2010).

History taking also includes observation of the patient and attention should be paid to visual cues, as well as explicit spoken responses. It is possible that concerns will be raised regarding vulnerable adults and child protection issues during any interaction with the patient and non-verbal cues may trigger these concerns. The HCP should be aware of the local policy and guidance in relation to vulnerable adults and child protection to ensure prompt action is taken if the HCP is uneasy during or following an interaction. For example: when asking a child to sit on the accompanying adult's lap or knee for visual acuity – signs of fear or unusual compliance may be cause for further investigation. However it is quite normal for a child to be scared of the test but not usually the adult.

Further information can be obtained from **http://www.isa.homeoffice.gov.uk/** (last accessed 23.09.11) in relation to Protection of Vulnerable Adults, and the NSPCC 2010 provides guidance around the legislation surrounding Safeguarding Children available at: **http://www.nspcc.org.uk/Inform/research/questions/child_protection_legislation_in_the_uk_pdf_wdf48953.pdf** (last accessed 23.09.11). We hope you find these resources useful.

Patient Education

Every ophthalmic nurse becomes involved in educating patients to care for themselves at home at some point within their career. This may be to prepare a patient for long-term eyedrop treatment which requires adherence and persistence, preparing a patient to manage their altered lifestyle due to sudden or gradual visual impairment or for short-term post operative care following ophthalmic surgery.

Davies (2006) suggests that the ophthalmic nurse has to develop lateral thinking when providing patient education particularly when discussing drop instillation. The home environment needs to be considered specifically around any physical limitations, lifestyle routines and timings for drops. The ophthalmic nurse may be faced with many challenges to support patients with drop instillation and in today's healthcare economy nurses from primary care cannot be relied upon to deliver post operative eyedrops.

Over the years, the ophthalmic nurse discovers from other nurses and patients themselvestips and tricks to help with drop instillation. Our advice would be to have a discussion among the experienced nurses to find out how they teach, what do they do and if it works. In all cases the patient must be supported to demonstrate how they would put in drops at home and encouraged to use appropriate techniques.

You may also be called upon to help a patient understand a specific condition. We encourage you to locate appropriate patient-friendly literature, have support telephone numbers available such as Sightline (01233 648170), a helpline provided by the International Glaucoma Association (http://www.glaucoma-association.com). You need to be able to access local contact numbers for patients to provide support strategies that they can use when they go home. A contact number for the ophthalmic outpatient department is always useful but you need to act according to your local guidelines and policies. We would advise talking to the experienced nurses within your unit about patient support.

The most important aspect of patient education is empowering your patient to understand their condition and to encourage them to take ownership of managing their condition in partnership with their doctor/HCP. This is the foundation for patient concordance with treatment. An effective communicator promotes this partnership approach and the ophthalmic nurse is often the first port of call for patients who need further explanations and clarification of information received about their condition.

Visual Acuity Testing

Visual Acuity Testing

History

Visual acuity testing was advised as long ago as 1843 when standardised vision testing charts were developed. Eduard von Jaeger published a set of reading samples to document functional vision in 1854. In 1861 Franciscus Donders, a Dutch ophthalmologist who was internationally regarded as an authority on eye diseases first used the term visual acuity describing visual precision. He defined it as the ratio between a patient's vision and standard vision.

Hermann Snellen published his famous chart in 1862. His most significant decision was not to use existing typefaces but to design unique figures called optotypes and based on a 5x5 grid. The grid was crucial because it was a physical standard measure to reproduce the chart. In 1875 the use of meters was introduced and this is why we have 6/6 in Britain and Europe, while in America feet continues to be the standard, therefore 20/20 is used to identify 'normal' vision.

Over the years a variety of questions were raised about Snellen's 'normal' vision. In 1898 Marius Tscherning explained Snellen's mistake that 20/20 does not represent the normal threshold for vision. Many individuals can read beyond Snellen's 'normal' as demonstrated in most units today but strangely the myth of 20/20 vision still exists. In 1959 Sloan designed different optotypes using 10 non-serif letters to be shown on each and every line to reduce the problem that not all letters are equally recognised (Colenbrander 2001).

John Green proposed a chart with geometric progression letter size in 1868 when working with both Donders and Snellen; however this new visual acuity testing grid was not accepted until 1976 when Bailey and Lovie published a new chart using five letters on each row with the spacing between the letters and rows being equal to the letter size. This ensured that the only variable on the chart was the letter size. This created an inverted triangle being wider at the top than the base following Green's idea of geometric progression for the letter sizes. In 1982 the National Eye Institute chose the Bailey–Lovie layout to establish a standardised method of testing and recording visual acuity for the Early Treatment of Diabetic Retinopathy study (NEI, 1999).

Alternative methods

In 1970 Dr Margaret Sheridan and Dr Peter Gardiner published an article in the British Medical Journal outlining the Sheridan–Gardiner vision screening test for school aged children and handicapped children of all ages (Sheridan & Gardiner, 1970). In 1976 Lea Hyvarinen created a chart using figures to measure acuity in pre-school children. This picture testing was regarded as inaccurate until Hazel Kay developed a picture test, supported by evidence based research, which proved that the pictures she produced could measure visual acuity in the same way the Snellen chart does for adults. In 1976, Hugh Taylor used the design principle from Lea to develop a 'Tumbling E Chart' for illiterates, which was used to study the visual acuity of Australian Aborigines.

In 1917 Dr Shinobu Ishihara published his red–green colour vision plates. The plates contain a circle of dots random in colour and size with a central pattern forming a number to individuals with normal colour vision. It is difficult to see or invisible for individuals with a red–green defect. The full test consists of 38 plates, but the existence of a deficiency is usually clear after a few plates. Testing the first 24 plates gives a more accurate diagnosis of the severity of the colour vision defect. Protanopia is the term used for those with an absence of long-wavelength sensitive retinal cones. Those with this condition are unable to distinguish between colours in the green–yellow–red section of the spectrum. Another condition called Deuteranopia also causes an inability to distinguish between colours in the green–yellow–red section of the spectrum.

Purpose

Visual acuity testing using a Snellen chart will have been practised for 150 years in 2012 and it is the initial procedure that all nurses working in an ophthalmic department and/or with patients with eye conditions will be expected to perform. This is for a number of reasons.

The healthcare professional examining the patient needs an objective baseline measurement for a patient's vision. This will enable the clinician to assess visual function at the patient's initial visit in the hospital eye service and clinical treatment decisions may, in part, be made due to the level of visual acuity, so it is a vital step in the process of accurate diagnosis for the patient (Marsden, 2007).

For example: the difference between Counting Fingers (CF) vision and 6/60 vision may influence the ability of a clinician to apply for funding for patients with wet macular degeneration (if LogMAR chart not available). A patient with CF vision is ineligible for Lucentis injections but a patient with 3/60 may meet the eligibility criteria. Moving the patient forward metre by metre as is outlined within this standard will achieve an accurate visual acuity documented within the patient record.

There are a variety of Snellen charts available and you must ensure that you are aware of the type of chart available in your unit. For example: Snellen is available as a 6m chart for use without a mirror and those of similar size designed to use with a mirror. Look at the letters; they are reversed to appear normal in the mirrored image.

The healthcare professional will also use the accurate visual acuity records to identify whether the patient has experienced an improvement in their vision or if their condition has deteriorated.

For example: following cataract surgery the healthcare professional will utilise the visual acuity record to identify initial improvement in vision. This does not replace an accurate refraction but gives an impression of the successful achievement of expected surgical outcomes.

The standards below outline the benchmarks for carrying out the following procedures:

Snellen chart visual acuity test

Sheridan–Gardiner visual acuity test

E cube visual acuity test

Kay Picture visual acuity test

LogMAR visual acuity test

Near vision test

Ishihara colour test

SNELLEN CHART VISUAL ACUITY

Standard Statement

Each patient will have an accurate assessment of distance vision recorded in medical notes precisely to aid ophthalmic examination and diagnosis.

Structure

The following resources are required:

- Adequate knowledge and skill to perform VA testing using Snellen chart (learner to be supervised by competent practitioner)
- Snellen chart
- Pinhole occluder
- Good lighting
- Patient's medical records
- Hard surface disinfectant according to local policy
- Box of tissues.

Process

The HCP should complete the following steps:

Introduce yourself to the patient, check the identity of the patient and explain the procedure.
To ensure the patient is correctly identified against the medical records and promote the patient's understanding in order to gain cooperation, obtain consent and allay anxiety.

Position the patient comfortably either sitting or standing at the distance equivalent to 6m from the Snellen chart.
To maintain correct position and to ensure comfort throughout the procedure.

Ensure good lighting of the chart and the environment.
To ensure accurate recording of visual acuity.

Establish whether the patient needs or has refractive correction for distance vision and correct where necessary, e.g. ask the patient to wear his/her distance spectacles. An alternative question could be to ask the patient to wear their driving or TV glasses if used. The use of refractive aids must be noted in the patient's record, including glasses or contact lenses.
To ensure that the patient's optimal vision is recorded.

Ask the patient to read the consecutive lines of letters from the Snellen chart diminishing in size using each eye in turn. The fellow eye is occluded with a clean occluder. It is possible to ask the patient to cover one eye at a time if the occluder is unavailable but care must be taken to ensure the patient does not depress the cornea of the fellow eye which would alter the vision in the covered eye when tested (Field, 2009). Write the result in the patient's medical record.
To assess the patient's visual acuity of each eye separately.

If the patient is unable to achieve a standard of 6/60 vision, he/she is walked forward towards the

Snellen chart, 1m at a time until the largest letter is seen with the tested eye. (Ensure you are able to measure 1m so that patient is moved forward appropriately. Local solutions will apply.)

To ensure the patient's optimal vision is recorded in their records.

The vision is recorded at the distance from which the largest letter is seen, e.g. 3/60 = 3m from the Snellen chart.

To assess vision precisely.

If a standard of 1/60 is not achieved, the patient is asked to count the number of fingers held up by the nurse in front of the affected eye, at varying distances less than one metre.

To record a visual acuity of counting fingers (CF).

If a standard of CF is not achieved, waving movements of the nurse's hands in front of the affected eye is performed.

To record visual acuity of hand movements (HM).

If HM is not achieved, light from a torch is shone toward the affected eye from four directions of a quadrant.

To record a visual acuity of perception of light (PL) and to determine in which part of the visual field light is perceived.

This is recorded in the following way:

X/PL

PL/X

If the patient can identify letters from the Snellen chart but does not achieve 6/6, i.e. normal vision, he/she should be tested with the pinhole occluder. The patient is asked to repeat the procedure above with the pinhole occluder in front of the affected eye at a distance of 6m only. (The unaffected eye is occluded at the same time.)

The structure and function of the retina is organised in such a way that fine visual acuity is produced in the central macular area. The use of the pinhole occluder reduces the peripheral rays of light going through the pupil area. It allows only a narrow bundle of rays to enter along the optical axis. It thus enables an assessment of central vision.

On completion of the procedure, the occluder should be disinfected according to local policy.

Note: The learner must always adhere to the usual infection control procedures within each department if different from the above information.

To eliminate cross infection.

Outcomes

The patient will:

    be able to understand, consent and cooperate with the test

    have an accurate visual acuity recorded in the medical records

    have a visual acuity history within the medical records.

SHERIDAN–GARDINER VISUAL ACUITY

Standard Statement

Each patient who has communication difficulties will have an accurate assessment of distance vision recorded in medical notes precisely to aid ophthalmic examination and diagnosis.

Structure

The following resources are required:

- Adequate knowledge and skill to perform VA testing using Sheridan–Gardiner chart (learner to be supervised by competent practitioner)
- Sheridan–Gardiner chart and letter identification cards
- Pinhole occluder
- Good lighting
- Patient's medical records
- Hard surface disinfectant according to local policy
- Box of tissues.

Process

The HCP should complete the following steps:

Introduce yourself to the patient, check the identity of the patient and explain the procedure.
To ensure the patient is correctly identified against the medical records and promote the patient's understanding in order to gain cooperation, obtain consent and allay anxiety.

Position the patient comfortably either sitting or standing at the distance equivalent to 6m from the nurse holding the Sheridan–Gardiner chart.
To maintain correct position and to ensure comfort throughout the procedure.

Ensure good lighting of the chart and the environment.
To ensure accurate recording of visual acuity.

Establish whether the patient needs or has refractive correction for distance vision and correct where necessary, e.g. ask the patient to wear his/her distance spectacles. An alternative question could be to ask the patient to wear their driving or TV glasses if used. The use of refractive aids must be noted in the patient's record, including glasses or contact lenses.
To ensure that the patient's optimal vision is recorded.

A nurse must supervise the following actions ensuring the fellow eye is occluded.
To ensure an accurate visual acuity is recorded for each eye.

The patient is asked to look at the letters on the Sheridan–Gardiner chart held by the examiner. Patient is asked to point on the letter identification card to the appropriate (same) letter as shown on the examiner's chart.

To assess the patient's visual acuity of each eye separately.

The fact that the Sheridan–Gardiner test has been used should be recorded in the patient's medical records.

To communicate the method of assessment to other relevant members of the healthcare team.

If the patient is unable to achieve a standard of 6/60 vision, the chart is brought forward one metre at a time until the largest letter can be seen. Proceed as for Recording Visual Acuity using Snellen chart.

For precise measurement of visual acuity.

On completion of the procedure, the occluder should be disinfected according to local policy. Note: The learner must always adhere to the usual infection control procedures within each department if different from the above information.

To eliminate cross infection.

Outcomes

The patient will:

 be able to understand and be able to cooperate with the test as fully as possible

 have an accurate visual acuity recorded in the medical records

 have a visual acuity history within the medical records.

E CUBE VISUAL ACUITY TEST

Standard Statement

Each patient who has communication difficulties will have an accurate assessment of distance vision recorded in medical notes precisely to aid ophthalmic examination and diagnosis.

Structure

The following resources are required:

- Adequate knowledge and skill to perform VA testing using E cube (Learner to be supervised by competent practitioner)
- E cube test
- Pinhole occluder
- Good lighting
- Patient's medical records
- Hard surface disinfectant according to local policy
- Box of tissues.

Process

The HCP should complete the following steps:

Introduce yourself to the patient, check the identity of the patient and explain the procedure.
To ensure the patient is correctly identified against the medical records and promote the patient's understanding in order to gain cooperation, obtain consent and allay anxiety.

Position the patient comfortably either sitting or standing holding the E shape at the distance equivalent to 6 m from the nurse holding the E cube (the E shape can be held showing different directions).
To maintain correct position and to ensure comfort throughout the procedure.

Ensure good lighting of the cube and the environment.
To ensure accurate recording of visual acuity.

Establish whether the patient needs or has refractive correction for distance vision and correct where necessary, e.g. ask the patient to wear his/her distance spectacles. An alternative question could be to ask the patient to wear their driving or TV glasses if used. The use of refractive aids must be noted in the patient's record, including glasses or contact lenses.
To ensure that the patient's optimal vision is recorded.

Another nurse must supervise the following actions ensuring the fellow eye is occluded.
To ensure an accurate visual acuity is recorded for each eye.

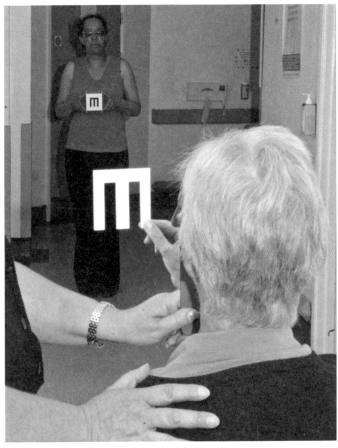

Figure 1

The patient is asked to look at the direction of the E held by the examiner and is asked to hold the E shape, turning it to the same way up as shown by the examiner (see Figure 1).

To assess the patient's visual acuity of each eye separately.

The fact that the E cube has been used should be recorded in the patient's medical records.

To communicate the method of assessment to other relevant members of the healthcare team.

If the patient is unable to achieve a standard of 6/60 vision, the examiner holding the E cube moves forward one metre at a time until the direction of the largest E can be seen. Proceed as for Recording Visual Acuity using Snellen Chart.

For precise measurement of visual acuity.

On completion of the procedure, the occluder should be disinfected according to local policy. Note: The learner must always adhere to the usual infection control procedures within each department if different from the above information.

To eliminate cross infection.

The tumbling E may also be found on a Snellen chart panel.

Outcomes

The patient will:
- understand and be able to cooperate with the test as fully as possible
- have an accurate visual acuity recorded in the medical records
- have a visual acuity history within the medical records.

KAY PICTURE VISUAL ACUITY TEST

Standard Statement

Each child will have an accurate assessment of visual acuity as soon as speech and naming ability is present – approximately 2 years of age using Kay Picture Test.

Structure

The following resources are required:

- Adequate knowledge and skill to perform VA testing using Kay Picture Test (learner to be supervised by competent practitioner)
- Kay Picture booklet and chart
- Eye patch and Micropore tape if occluder cannot be used.
- Pinhole occluder
- Good lighting
- Patient's medical records
- Hard surface disinfectant according to local policy
- Box of tissues.

Process

The HCP should complete the following steps:

Introduce yourself to the patient, check the identity of the patient and explain the procedure.
To ensure the patient is correctly identified against the medical records and promote the patient's understanding in order to gain cooperation, obtain consent and allay anxiety.

Position the child comfortably sitting at a distance equivalent to 6 m from the person holding the Kay Picture booklet. Usually sitting on accompanying adult's knee or lap.
To obtain the child's visual acuity accurately.

Ensure good lighting of chart and of environment.
To maintain child's correct position throughout procedure and accurate recording of VA.

Cover the child's left eye with patch if possible. Open booklet with numbered index on your right and use your right thumb to choose size and flick page over so that the chosen picture faces the child.
To present the child with a specific picture at the identified size.

Begin with a large picture and ask the child to identify it, repeat showing smaller and smaller pictures until you have reach smallest size child can see and identify clearly. Always give lots of praise and encouragement during the process.
To ensure optimal VA is identified and ensuring the child is having fun during the procedure – to gain cooperation and reduce anxiety.

Repeat the process covering the right eye if possible.
To ensure accurate assessment of both eyes.

Record VA in the same manner as recording using a Snellen chart, i.e. 6/36, 6/12 in the patient's record.

To comply with legal requirements and communicate with other healthcare professionals regarding method used for assessment.

Outcomes

The child will

understand why the procedure is necessary and be able to cooperate

be able to cooperate and perform the test accurately

have an accurate visual acuity recorded in the medical records.

LogMAR VISUAL ACUITY TEST

Each patient will have an accurate assessment of distance vision recorded in medical notes precisely to aid ophthalmic examination and diagnosis and meet medico/legal requirements using LogMAR vision chart.

Structure

The following resources are required:

- Nurses with adequate knowledge and competence
- LogMAR chart (there are different distance charts available – ensure you are aware of the correct distance for the chart used in your department and adjust the standard accordingly)
- Plain/pinhole occluder
- Box of tissues
- Hard surface disinfectant according to local policy
- Good lighting
- Patient's medical records
- Understanding of recording LogMAR VA in medical records:

    LogMAR charts are designed to be used at 4m distance.

    Top line = 1.0

    Each line below will give a score of 0.1 less than the line above.

    Each letter in each line scores 0.02

    If patient reads the whole of 0.4 line score = 0.4

    If patient reads the whole of 0.4 + 3 letters from 0.3 the score is 0.36.

    Some units document the number of letters read from the LogMAR chart.

    For example, if the patient reads to 0.4 plus three letters from 0.3, the score would be 38 (0.4 = 35 letters plus 3 from 0.3). Please document your scores according to local policy.

Process

The HCP should complete the following steps:

Introduce yourself to the patient, check the identity of the patient and explain the procedure.

To ensure the patient is correctly identified against the medical records and promote the patient's understanding in order to gain cooperation, obtain consent and allay anxiety.

Position the patient comfortably either sitting or standing at the distance equivalent to 4m from the LogMAR chart. Note: different size charts need different distances [may be 4m, 2m or 1m].

To maintain correct position and to ensure comfort throughout the procedure.

Ensure good lighting of the chart and the environment.

To ensure accurate recording of visual acuity.

Establish whether the patient needs refractive correction for distance vision and correct where necessary, e.g. ask the patient to wear his/her spectacles. The use of refractive aids must be noted in the patient's record.

To ensure that the patient's optimal vision is recorded.

Ask the patient to read from the LogMAR chart the consecutive lines of letters that diminish in size – each eye in turn is occluded. Note the result in the patient's record.

To assess the patient's visual acuity of each eye separately.

If the patient is unable to achieve a standard of 1.0 vision, either move the chart or the patient forward to a distance of 1m. The vision is recorded by adding 0.6 to the LogMAR.

To assess vision precisely.

If unable to read any letters from LogMAR chart at 1m then use another means of visual assessment.

Repeat the process for the other eye.

To ensure accurate visual acuity is recorded in the patient record

On completion of the procedure, the occluder should be disinfected according to local policy. Note: The learner must always adhere to the usual infection control procedures within each department if different from the above information.

To eliminate cross infection.

Outcomes

The patient will:

understand and be able to cooperate with the test

have an accurate visual acuity recorded in the medical records

have a visual acuity history recorded within the medical records.

NEAR VISION TESTING

Standard Statement

Each patient will have the near vision test to establish how well the patient can see to read at close range.

Structure

The following resources are required:

- Adequate knowledge and skill to perform near vision testing (learner to be supervised by competent practitioner)
- Near vision reading booklet
- Patient's reading spectacles if required
- Pinhole occluder
- Good lighting
- Patient's medical records
- Hard surface disinfectant according to local policy
- Box of tissues.

Process

The HCP should complete the following steps:

Introduce yourself to the patient, check the identity of the patient and explain the procedure.

To ensure the patient is correctly identified against the medical records and promote the patient's understanding in order to gain cooperation, obtain consent and allay anxiety.

The patient should use their reading glasses if necessary.

To obtain best corrected vision during the near vision test.

Seat the patient comfortably and instruct the patient to hold the test type booklet at a comfortable reading distance.

To maintain correct position throughout the procedure

Ask the patient to cover one eye. This may be with an occluder or the patient may feel more comfortable cupping one hand over the fellow eye. Note: ensure a cupped hand is used or the patient may compress the cornea altering fellow eye vision when tested. If an occluder is used, ensure it is cleaned according to local policy to prevent cross infection.

To check the reading vision from a single eye.

Keep normal room lights on (do not include additional light source unless the patient indicates that this is their usual practice).

To ascertain their normal reading vision.

The patient should then be asked to indicate the smallest print they can read comfortably.

NB the smallest print type is N5 and as the number increases the print becomes larger up to N45.

To ascertain their ability to read print.

Each eye is checked individually as with Snellen distance vision and both eyes are recorded in the patient's record

To ensure accurate measurement and recording of near vision test (NMC, 2010).

To communicate the method of assessment with other healthcare professionals.

Outcomes

The patient will:

understand what is happening and be able to cooperate with the procedure

be able to cooperate and perform the test accurately

have an accurate near vision test for both eyes recorded in medical notes to aid diagnosis.

ISHIHARA COLOUR VISION TEST

Standard Statement

All patients presenting with suspected optic nerve abnormality will have documented assessment of their colour vision using an Ishihara Colour-Vision Test. 38 Plate edition.

Structure

The following resources are required:

- Adequate knowledge and skill to perform near vision testing (learner to be supervised by competent practitioner)
- The series of plates designed as a test for colour blindness by Shinobu Ishihara
- A room lit adequately by natural daylight.

Process

The HCP should complete the following steps:

Introduce yourself to the patient, check the identity of the patient and explain the procedure.
To ensure the patient is correctly identified against the medical records and promote the patient's understanding in order to gain cooperation, obtain consent and allay anxiety.

Position patient comfortably in a chair in a room lit by natural daylight or reasonable light source if twilight/evening. Document time in patient records.
The use of electric light may produce some discrepancy in the results because of an alteration in the appearance of shades of colour.

Hold Ishihara plates 75 cm from the patient, tilted so that the plane of the paper is at right angles to the line of vision.
Patient is able to see plates fully.

Cover one eye fully using occluder.
Each eye will be tested independently to ascertain which eye has abnormality.

Ask the patient to say which number they can see on the plate. Each answer should ideally be given with not more than three seconds delay.
Patient has adequate time to perceive colour and respond.

If the patient is unable to read numbers use plates 26–38 which have winding coloured lines, which should be traced within ten seconds.
Patient has adequate time to perceive colour and respond

If 17 or more plates are read normally the colour vision is regarded as normal and should be documented as 'Ishihara full' or Ishihara 17/17.
Normal colour vision measurement is accurately documented.

If only 13 or fewer plates are read as normal, colour vision is regarded as deficient and should be documented as 'n'/17 Ishihara, where n is the number of plates read.

Abnormal colour vision measurement is accurately documented and as such reported.

Occlude fellow eye and repeat procedure.

Both eyes are measured.

On completion of the procedure, the occluder should be disinfected according to local policy. Note: The learner must always adhere to the usual infection control procedures within each department if different from the above information.

To eliminate cross infection.

Outcomes

The patient will:

understand, consent and cooperate with procedure

have the best opportunity to perceive shades of colour accurately

be informed of how to perform test to ensure accurate outcome

have colour-vision assessment recorded in the medical records.

Ocular Medications

Ocular Medications

History

Ocular medications have been available for many centuries and are used to treat a number of eye disorders or as a diagnostic tool. In 3000 BC the Chinese distilled the mahuang plant, which contains ephedrine hydrochloride and was used as a decongestant. Today, in some countries ephedrine hydrochloride is still used to treat minor eye irritations.

In India, approximately 120–162 AD, a physician called Charaka was using eye drops to treat various ailments and in medieval times, the Italians used drops prepared from the belladonna plant to dilate women's pupils, an effect considered attractive. Bella Donna translates in Italian as beautiful lady. Belladonna drops acted as an anticholinergic agent, blocking receptors in the muscles of the eye that constrict pupil size. Today atropine, which mimics the same effect, has been purified from the belladonna plant since the 1830s.

In the 1900s cocaine was brought to Europe from America. The active component of coca leaves, namely cocaine, was extracted and Karl Koller demonstrated the possibility of using cocaine as a viable method of anaesthetizing the eye in 1884. This drug was still being used in the 1980s to test for Horner's syndrome whereby these drops blocked the reuptake of norepinephrine resulting in dilation of the pupil (provocation test) (Van der Wiel and Van Gijn, 1986). Kanski (2007) continues to describe the use of cocaine 4% but as safer drugs such as apraclonidine with fewer side effects have been developed it is very rarely used in the UK.

Ocular medication can be found either as a drop or ointment. Eye drops are basically medication contained within a watery solution. Ointments contain medication but within an oily solution. This is because the active medication needs to stay in contact with the globe or eyelids for a longer period for effective delivery of medication. Occasionally medications are slightly thicker than water, e.g. carbomers (Viscotears gel) and are provided in a tube.

Eye drops and the Healthcare Assistant

Most eye drops used in the ophthalmic setting are prescription only medicines (POM) and as such, are regulated by the Medicines Act 1968. POM administration is restricted to suitable practitioner, e.g. a registered nurse. However Marsden (2007) explains that administration of POM eyedrops can be undertaken by a non-registered nurse (healthcare assistant) as these medicines are categorised as non-parenteral (topical) and are therefore exempt by the Prescription Only Medicines (Human Use) Order 1997, Article 9 (http://www.legislation.gov.uk/uksi/1997/1830/article/9/made Last accessed 16.10.11).

Anatomy and Physiology

The healthcare professional (HCP) should be aware of the composition of tears as it is a medium for the absorption of ocular medications.

The tear film consists of three layers:

1. The mucoid layer lies adjacent to the corneal epithelium. It improves the wetting properties of the tears. It is produced by the goblet cells in the conjunctival epithelium.

2. The aqueous (watery) layer is produced by the main lachrymal gland in the supero-temporal part of the orbit and accessory lacrimal glands found in the conjunctival stroma. This aqueous layer contains electrolytes, proteins, lysozyme, immunoglobulin, glucose and dissolved oxygen (from the atmosphere).

3. The oily layer (superficial layer of the tear film produced by meibomian glands – modified sebaceous gland) of the eyelid margins. This oily layer helps maintain the vertical column of tears between the upper and lower lids and prevents excessive evaporation.

Ocular medications are used for a variety of reasons by ophthalmic healthcare professionals.

As an aid to diagnosis or treatment:

- To dilate pupil as a means of examining or photographing the posterior segment or retina within a clinic setting.
- For patients needing cataract surgery.
- Dyes (drops or strips) to aid the healthcare professional using a slit lamp for corneal and dendrite ulcers, foreign bodies etc.
- To anaesthetise an eye to examine.

As a treatment for various ocular disorders:

- Glaucoma.
- Allergic reactions.
- Lubrication.
- Infections.
- Inflammations.
- Post operative treatment (e.g. following cataract, retinal, ocular plastic surgery)
- Cycloplegic refraction counteracting the effects of accommodation in children to obtain an accurate refraction. The pupil response is absent with dilating eye drops excluding the child's natural high level of accommodation.

Important note

Tears normally flow away through a drainage system formed by the puncta (inferior and superior), canaliculus (inferior and superior), the common canaliculus, opening into the lacrimal sac, the nasolacrimal duct (which drains into the nose). To stop systemic absorption of some ocular medication, especially those used to treat the glaucomas and ocular hypertension, patients should be taught to occlude the lower puncta after instilling drops.

The HCP should be aware that eye drops can cause inflammation or even sting as there are active elements. In extreme cases, patients can develop or present with symptoms of dizziness, confusion, tachycardia, and difficulty swallowing. Patients should be monitored after instillation and any side effects should be recorded. An example is using dilatation eyedrops such as Tropicamide 1% which will dilate the pupil. This in turn reduces the width of the drainage angle and may raise the intraocular pressure in individuals with shallow anterior chambers. The HCP should be aware of the potential side effects of all eyedrops administered within the clinic or supplied as a take home drug.

The HCP must make sure that if patients are using contact lenses, they are removed before instilling drops.

INSTILLATION OF DILATING EYE DROPS

Standard Statement

All patients will have their dilating eye drops administered safely without risk of cross infection or adverse reactions.

Structure

The following resources are required:

- Adequate knowledge and skill to instil eye drops (learner to be supervised by a competent practitioner)
- Relevant eye drops
- Prescription chart/valid prescription within patient's own medical records
- Tissues
- Access to facilities for hand washing.
- Pen torch to check for relative afferent pupillary defect (RAPD) and anterior chamber (AC) depth assessment if instilling dilating drops.

Process

The HCP should complete the following steps:

Introduce yourself to the patient, check the identity of the patient and explain the procedure.
To ensure the patient is correctly identified against the medical records and promote the patient's understanding in order to gain cooperation, obtain consent and allay anxiety.

Explain to the patient why the ophthalmologist needs to view the retina at the back of the eye during the consultation.
This is to facilitate an accurate assessment of the retinal structures and to ensure the patient understands why the drops are needed.

Explain why it is not safe to drive for 4–6 hours following dilating drops due to altered visual function.
To ensure patient understands risks following eye drop instillation.

Check with patient and notes for known allergies to medications/eye drops and document any findings in patient's notes.
To reduce risk of adverse reactions and promote communication between patient and the HCP.

Carry out the procedure for checking pupils for relative afferent pupillary defect (RAPD)
To identify any abnormality prior to instillation of drops.

Wash and dry hands thoroughly.
The HCP should follow own organisation's infection control policy on hand washing to reduce the risk of cross infection.

Ensure patient is positioned comfortably with head well supported.
To ensure comfort and reduce movement of head during instillation

Check the name of the patient against the prescription within the patient's medical records or prescription chart. Check the prescription of the eye drops applies to the correct patient.

To ensure that the correct patient receives the correct eye drops.

Give patient a clean tissue if patient is able to hold it.

To prevent cross infection to the nose or other eye.

Stand so that your dominant hand rests gently on the patient's forehead.

To prevent the eye dropper or tip of bottle from touching the eye, lids or lashes.

Ask the patient to look up to the ceiling gently extending neck if possible.
Pull the lower lid down gently with other hand.

The drop will fall into the lower fornix and prevent blinking, which occurs if the drop falls onto the cornea.

Instil one drop into the lower fornix without touching the eye, the lids or lashes with the eye dropper or tip of bottle.

Only one drop will be held in the eye, as additional drops will spill over the lid margins. No contact will prevent cross infection.

Ask patient to relax neck and gently close the eye avoiding the tendency to squeeze the eye closed.

This will allow time for absorption of drops.

The patient can gently wipe away any excess drops with the clean tissue if able.

For the patient's comfort and prevent possible skin irritation.

Dispose of the tissue for the patient in the nearest clinical waste bin. Offer another tissue for second eye if both eyes have to be dilated.

To prevent cross infection.

Sign prescription with date, time and print name following signature.

To indicate when drops have been given and who has given the drops.

For the unregistered HCP, ensure you follow local guidelines which may include obtaining a countersignature from the registered nurse for administration of eyedrop POM.

Outcomes

The patient will:

understand and consent to dilating eye drops administered
understand the risks and benefits of dilating the pupils
have correct eye drops instilled safely without risk of cross infection.

Common abbreviations are: G. Gutt., Guttae = Drops

TEACHING PATIENTS TO INSTIL EYE DROPS

All patients will be taught to self medicate eyedrops safely without risk of cross infection if both eyes have prescribed topical medications

Structure

The following resources are required:

- Adequate knowledge and skill to teach instillation of eye drops (learner to be supervised by a competent practitioner)
- Relevant eye drops
- Prescription chart/valid prescription within patient's own medical records
- Tissues
- Access to facilities for hand washing for patient and the HCP.

Process

The HCP should complete the following steps:

Introduce yourself to the patient, check the identity of the patient and explain the procedure.
To ensure the patient is correctly identified against the medical records and promote the patient's understanding in order to gain cooperation, obtain consent and allay anxiety.

Explain to the patient why they need to use eyedrops as a treatment.
This is to provide an accurate assessment of the patient's ability to see properly and to ensure patient understands why the drops are needed.

Explain why it is not safe to drive if part of their treatment is the instillation of dilating drops as they will suffer from altered visual function. If using multiple drops advise to leave at least 10 minutes between each drop. If ointment is also part of their treatment, instruct to instil last.
To ensure patient understands risks following eye drop instillation. Spreading the instillation of each drop will ensure optimum absorption of each drop. Ointment will create a barrier, drops will not be absorbed.

Check with patient and notes for known allergies to medications/eye drops and document any findings in patient's notes.
To reduce risk of adverse reactions and promote communication between patient and the HCP.

Ask the patient to wash and dry hands thoroughly and advise to continue this practice at home.
To reduce the risk of cross infection.

Ensure patient is positioned comfortably with head well supported.
To ensure comfort and reduce movement of head during instillation.

Ensure that clean tissues are within reach for the patient to use.
To prevent cross infection to the nose or other eye.

Ensure seal around the top of bottle has not been broken if it is a new bottle. Give bottle to patient and ensure that patient can break seal. Ask patient to remove top and place on clean surface.

To reduce the risk of cross infection. To ensure that patient can remove seal from future bottles if treatment will continue after first bottle.

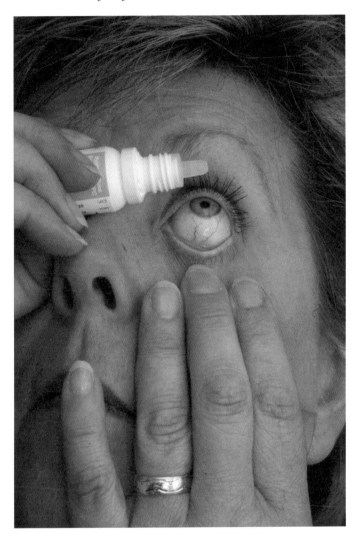

Figure 2

Ask the patient to look up to the ceiling gently extending neck if possible. Ask the patient to balance the bottle of drops on the bridge of their nose with their dominant hand. Ask the patient to pull the lower lid down gently with other hand creating a 'well' (see Figure 2)

The drop will fall into the lower fornix and prevent blinking, which occurs if the drop falls onto the cornea.

Instruct the patient to squeeze the bottle. This will instil one drop into the lower fornix without touching the eye, the lids or lashes with the eye dropper or tip of bottle.

Only one drop will be held in the eye, as additional drops will spill over the lid margins. No contact will prevent cross infection.

NB *Some eyedrop bottles have different methods of delivery – some tap the base of the bottle, some squeeze the button on the side of the bottle. Be aware of the delivery method for each individual bottle and adapt the instructions appropriately.*

Ask patient to relax neck and gently close the eye avoiding the tendency to squeeze the eye closed.

This will allow time for absorption of drops.

If the patient has difficulty holding the bottle across the bridge of the nose, this alternative method can be tried.

To facilitate alternative methods to support patient adherence.

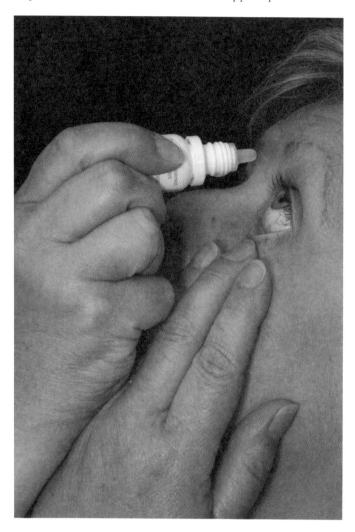

Figure 3

Ask the patient to hold the bottle in their dominant hand and place their other hand flat on the cheek, gently pulling their lower lid downwards creating a 'well' with their fingertips. The dominant hand, holding the bottle can then be placed on top of the other hand with the tip of the eyedrop bottle visible in front of the eye but not dipping towards the cornea. Ask the patient to look up, gently extend the neck and using the appropriate delivery method allow one drop to fall into the eye (see Figure 3).

The drop will fall into the eye without contact with the globe and reduce risk of cross infection.

If the patient has difficulty in extending the neck suggest lying down or leaning backwards.
To promote correct positioning.

If the patient has physical difficulty, e.g. poor dexterity or finger strength, due to co-morbidities such as arthritis preventing the delivering of one drop, eyedrop instillation aids are available from most pharmaceutical companies.

Alternative methods of drop instillation must be explored with the patient to ensure optimal treatment is provided. It cannot be assumed that community services will provide eyedrop instillation so please check your local agreements.

Facilitate safe disposal of the tissue for the patient in the nearest clinical waste bin. Ensure that clean tissues are available for second eye if both eyes have to be treated. Repeat the process again for second eye.

To prevent cross infection.

Ask the patient to take note of the date that treatment commenced as expiry date will be 28 days after this.

This is to provide an accurate assessment of the patient's ability to understand why a new eye drops bottle must commence after 28 days even if the current drop bottle is not empty.

Remind patients to obtain further supplies of their eye drop treatment from their GP before their current bottle expires or runs out.

To ensure continuity of treatment if required.

Document that patient has been instructed on how to use eye drops and has been observed using eye drops safely according to local policy.

To provide full documentation of the care episode in the medical records.

For the unregistered HCP, ensure you follow local guidelines which may include obtaining a countersignature from a registered nurse for administration of eye drop POM

Outcomes

The patient will:
    understand and consent to having eye drops
    understand the risks and benefits
    have correct eye drops instilled safely without risk of cross infection.

Common abbreviations are: G. Gutt., Guttae = Drops

TEACHING PATIENTS TO INSTIL EYE OINTMENT

Standard Statement

All patients will be taught to self administer eye ointment safely without risk of cross infection if both eyes are prescribed topical medications.

Structure

The following resources are required:

- Adequate knowledge and skill to teach application of eye ointment (learner to be supervised by a competent practitioner)
- Relevant eye ointment
- Prescription chart/valid prescription within patient's own medical records
- Tissues
- Access to facilities for hand washing for HCP and patient.

Process

The HCP should complete the following steps:

Introduce yourself to the patient, check the identity of the patient and explain the procedure.
To ensure the patient is correctly identified against the medical records and promote the patient's understanding in order to gain cooperation, obtain consent and allay anxiety.

Explain to the patient why the ophthalmologist needs to use this method as a treatment.
This is to provide an accurate assessment of the patient's ability to understand why the ointment is needed and not drops.

Explain why it is not safe to drive for at least 5 minutes following the instillation of ointment(s) due to altered visual function.
To ensure patient understands risks following eye ointment instillation.

Check with patient and medical notes for known allergies to medications, eye drops, ointment or wool and document any findings in patient's notes. Alert the clinician to wool allergies.
To reduce risk of adverse reactions and promote communication between patient and the HCP.
Note: many ointments have wool fat as a component and can cause allergic reactions.

Ask the patient to wash and dry hands thoroughly and advise to continue this practice at home.
To reduce the risk of cross infection.

Ensure patient fully understands the process.
To gain consent for procedure, cooperation and ensure understanding.

Ensure that clean tissues are within reach for the patient to use.
To prevent cross infection to the nose or other eye.

Ensure seal around the top of ointment has not been broken if it is a new tube. Give ointment to patient and ensure that patient can break seal. Ask patient to remove top and place on clean surface.
To reduce the risk of cross infection. To ensure that patient can remove seal from future tubes of ointment if treatment will continue after the first tube.

Ask patient to use dominant hand to hold tube. Ask patient to use opposite hand to gently pull lower lid creating a 'well'. Ask patient to tilt head backwards and look up to the ceiling.

To aid a safe delivery of ointment to the globe.

To ensure that the tip of the tube will not touch the cornea during the delivery of the ointment.

The HCP should stand in front of the patient to assess that the 'well' has been created.

The HCP is assessing the patient for compliance and understanding.

Ask the patient to gently squeeze the ointment into the 'well' ensuring that the tip of the tube remains clear of the cornea. Instruct the patient to start at the nasal aspect and stop at the temporal aspect then close eyes before moving the tube away from the lids.

No contact will prevent cross infection. The cornea will not be touched by the tip of the tube.

Ask patient to relax neck and keep eye gently closed, avoiding the tendency to squeeze eye closed.

This will allow time for absorption of ointment.

The patient can gently wipe away any excess ointment with the clean tissue if able.

For the patient's comfort and prevent possible skin irritation.

Explain that the ointment may feel sticky until it melts into the globe.

To facilitate an understanding for the patient using this treatment.

Facilitate safe disposal of the tissue for the patient in the nearest clinical waste bin. Ensure that clean tissues are available for second eye if both eyes have to be treated. Repeat the process again for second eye.

To prevent cross infection.

Ask the patient to take note of the date that treatment commenced as expiry date will be 28 days after this.

This is to provide an accurate assessment of the patient's ability to understand why a new tube of ointment must commence after 28 days even if the current tube is not empty.

Document that patient has been instructed on how to use eye ointment and has been observed using eye ointment safely according to local policy.

To provide full documentation of the care episode in the medical records.

Note: Eye ointment may be used elsewhere on the eyelids or face. Ensure patient is observed applying the ointment to the appropriate area safely.

For the unregistered HCP, ensure you follow local guidelines which may include obtaining a countersignature from the registered nurse for application of eye ointment POM.

Outcomes

The patient will:

 understand and agree to administer own eye ointment

 understand the risks and benefits of using eye ointment

 demonstrate correct use of eye ointment and be able to self administer safely without risk of cross infection.

Common abbreviation is: Oc = Ointment

The Ophthalmic Outpatient Department

The Ophthalmic Outpatient Department

As the new nurse in ophthalmology, you will be using your newly acquired skills in visual acuity testing regardless of where you work in ophthalmology. These skills are the first steps for a new nurse in any ophthalmic setting. Once you have mastered testing the vision you will quickly progress to learning many new skills and the likely next steps will include history taking, assessment of the anterior chamber depth and identification of a relative afferent pupillary defect. Your pen torch is a most useful tool and can be used in many ways. Assessing the function of a variety of ocular structures is also the remit of the ophthalmic nurse, including the tear function by performing a Schirmer's test and macular function using the Amsler grid. However an accurate recording of the presenting condition and the past ophthalmic/medical history is the first action for all ophthalmic nurses. This information allows the nurse to decide which test or investigation is required for each individual patient as well as whether there are any identifiable contraindications to be considered.

Many nursing techniques such as pen torch assessment of anterior chamber depth have been developed to ensure patient safety prior to pupil dilatation. It is possible to artificially reduce the drainage angle during dilatation causing an increase in intraocular pressure when a patient has a narrow drainage angle (Elliott, 2003). The presence of a shallow anterior chamber may indicate a narrow drainage angle. Anterior chamber depth assessment is usually followed by assessing the patient for relative afferent pupillary defects, sometimes called Marcus-Gunn pupil. This test identifies abnormal optic nerve function. When looking for direct and consensual response the affected eye will not respond by constricting due to reduced light impulses being passed down the afferent pathway. A consensual response will be seen when the light is shown into the non-affected eye (Madge, 2006b).

The Schirmer's test has been practised for over 100 years and was originally developed in 1903 by Otto Schirmer. This is a basic test to measure tear function for an individual at a given time. This test measures quantity rather than the quality of tears. Marsden (2007) advises us that alternative methods of measuring tear film drainage such as specialist cameras are available. Yet until an alternative quick and inexpensive method is identified, the Schirmer's test is likely to continue to be carried out by ophthalmic nurses in nearly all ophthalmic outpatient departments.

The Amsler Grid as invented by Marc Amsler, a Swedish ophthalmologist, assesses macular function. This grid gives the ophthalmic nurse a tool to measure the central 10° visual field. This ensures the blind spot is outside of the area to be measured. It is a quick and easy measurement to assess for metamorphopsia (visual distortion). Some patients can be taught how to monitor their condition at home to ensure early changes in macular function are identified and this prompts the patient to seek appropriate help. This obviously relies on the ophthalmic nurse helping the patient to understand what the test is for and how to perform it at home (Elliott, 2003).

When the nurse has mastered these basic skills continuing to develop their knowledge and experience, it is likely that more advanced skills will be required such as nasolacrimal duct syringing. This test assesses the patency of the lacrimal drainage system and is often requested when patients complain of persistent watering eyes. Be aware that patients with facial palsies will often have watery eyes as this condition will often result in malposition of the punctum as will conditions such as entropion (turning of lid towards globe) and ectropion (turning of lid away from globe).

Most ophthalmic nurses will be required to either insert or remove bandage contact lenses. These lenses do not have any refractive power (Shaw *et al.*, 2010) and are used to provide a barrier between the cornea and the atmosphere similar to a plaster on a cut. Marsden (2007) explains that they are used to promote healing of a small corneal leak or to protect the cornea in conditions such as persistent epithelial defects.

Many ophthalmic outpatient departments will carry out fundus fluorescein angiography (FFA) testing and this is now often the remit of the ophthalmic nurse. FFA is a diagnostic test that identifies damage to or leakage from the retinal or choroidal circulation. Additional skills such as intravenous cannulation and drug administration are required to perform this test as well as taking informed consent therefore the ophthalmic nurse must be able to obtain a full medical history with emphasis on allergies to dyes and lung disorders such as asthma. Intravenous fluorescein itself can result in a severe anaphylactic reaction therefore the ophthalmic nurse must have the skills to provide immediate emergency support to the affected individual. Marsden (2007) explains that although the fluorescein itself does not affect the patient's blood pressure, the flashing light from rapid photography may result in vagal stimulation leading to bradycardia and hypotension. It is for this reason that many ophthalmic units require additional certificated skills in intermediate life support for nurses performing the FFA procedure. The new nurse to an ophthalmic outpatient department must be able to provide evidence that these advanced skills have been obtained and kept up to date according to the local unit policy.

All interventions and actions must be documented within the patient's medical record in accordance with the Nursing and Midwifery Council and guidance on record keeping which forms part of the holistic care for a patient (NMC, 2010).

HISTORY TAKING IN CLINIC

Standard Statement

All patients will have an accurate history taken and documented in clinical notes

Structure

The following resources are required:

- Adequate knowledge and skill to obtain an accurate history from the patient (learner to be supervised by competent practitioner)
- Patient Medical Notes
- Private area for assessment.

Process

The HCP should complete the following steps:

Introduce yourself to the patient, check the identity of the patient and explain the procedure.

To ensure the patient is correctly identified against the medical records and promote the patient's understanding in order to gain cooperation, obtain consent and allay anxiety.

Position the patient comfortably, ensuring privacy.

To promote cooperation and confidentiality.

Ask the patient why they have attended clinic today and review any referral letter from the GP and/ or optician noting primary referral reason.

To ensure all adequate preparation is carried out to provide effective and efficient patient flow within clinics e.g. dilatation of pupils if referred for a retinal condition.

Ask about previous personal ophthalmic history, e.g. eye operations.

To aid diagnosis identifying significant previous ophthalmic problems that might be relevant to this episode of care, e.g. previous corneal surgery or laser may affect the K readings taken prior to cataract surgery.

Ask about any known family ophthalmic problems such as glaucoma, unexplained blindness.

To identify any known risk factor linked to ophthalmic conditions such as glaucoma. Many ophthalmic conditions have familial traits or genetic predisposition and therefore these patients are more at risk of developing the disease themselves. However remember that family history is not always known and unexplained blindness can highlight unknown risk factors.

Ask about past or present medical problems and medication including over the counter preparations.

To ascertain if any medical problem or medication is related to an ophthalmic problem. For example: a history of diabetes, hypertension, thyroid disease, rheumatoid arthritis, Crohn's and spondylitis of the spine, CVA and/or TIA.

Medications like warfarin, oral steroids and some antidepressants have an ophthalmic effect as well as interactions with topical preparations that may be prescribed.

Ask about known allergies or reactions to foodstuffs and medications.

To identify any specific substance that should be avoided by a prescribing clinician.

Ask about social factors that may influence structure and function of both the eye and the whole body.

To establish risk factors of known ophthalmic disease such as smoking and macular degeneration, poor liver function in a heavy drinker, frequent attendance at Outpatients affecting employment and driving with poor visual acuity. These facts may influence the development of a suitable plan of care for the individual patient.

Record visual acuity as per standard of care.

To obtain baseline data and comply with legal requirements.

Examine the eye with pen torch in a systematic manner documenting abnormalities if found, checking anterior chamber depth and for relative afferent pupillary defect as per standards of care if dilatation is required.

To aid diagnosis, provide safe nursing interventions and provide the clinician with a complete history.

If necessary perform ocular hygiene as per standard of care.

To provide patient comfort and remove debris from ocular structures facilitating adequate examination.

All information should be documented in the patient's record.

To provide a clear record of nursing intervention and reduce repetition for the patient.

Patient and medical records will be taken to the appropriate clinic room and informed of any waiting time.

To ensure patient is seen by the correct clinician at the appropriate time or is kept informed of any unexpected delays.

Outcomes

The patient will:

understand what is happening and be able to cooperate with the procedure

not have to repeat information as full ophthalmic history is documented in medical notes

have any abnormality identified, documented and discussed with medical colleague before continuing with other procedures such as dilatation of pupils

be seen according to appointment with correct doctor

be kept informed of any delay to clinic running time.

PEN TORCH EXAMINATION

Standard Statement

All patients will have both eyes examined with a pen torch before any nursing intervention takes place.

Structure

The following resources are required:

- Adequate knowledge and skill to perform a pen torch assessment of the anterior chamber (learner to be supervised by competent practitioner)
- Pen torch with bright light
- Patient medical records
- Box of tissues
- Access to hand washing facilities.

Process

The HCP should complete the following steps:

Introduce yourself to the patient, check the identity of the patient and explain the procedure.
To ensure the patient is correctly identified against the medical records and promote the patient's understanding in order to gain cooperation, obtain consent and allay anxiety.

Wash and dry hands thoroughly.
To reduce the risk of cross contamination with microorganisms.

Observe the whole of the patient's face first and note any abnormalities in patient's record.
To identify any facial abnormalities that may interfere with ocular movement.

Eye examined systematically from the outside structures inwards towards the lens:
With patient's eyes closed examine:
Eyelids for:
- swelling
- discoloration/bruising
- discharge
- entropion
- ectropion.

With patient's eye open and asked to look up and down appropriately examine:
Conjunctiva for:
- injection (redness)
- subconjunctival haemorrhage
- chemosis (oedema)
- section: intact, suture line
- iris prolapse
- presence of bleb.

With patient looking straight ahead examine:

Cornea for:

- clarity (clear, hazy, cloudy), encroaching blood vessel.

Anterior chamber for:

- depth
- hypopyon
- hyphaema.

Iris for:

- peripheral iridotomy if you are able to visualize it.
- abnormal lesions.

Pupil for:

- shape (peaked, round)
- size (dilated, miosed)
- reaction
- position.

Lens for:

- intraocular lens (IOL) especially if anterior chamber lens is used.
- opacities
- dislocation of lens or IOL

All ocular structures are systematically examined using a pen torch light source. Always compare your findings to the fellow eye.

Document procedure in the patient's medical records.

To ensure accurate recording in patient's notes.

Dispose of non-reusable equipment and waste into a yellow waste bin according to Trust infection control guidelines.

To comply with policies and procedures of the organisation.

Outcomes

The patient will:

 understand and be able to cooperate with the investigation

 be comfortable and able to maintain position during the procedure

 not be exposed to the risk of cross infection.

ANTERIOR CHAMBER (AC) DEPTH ASSESSMENT

Standard Statement

All patients requiring dilatation during clinical examination will have the depth of the anterior chamber assessed and all patients with shallow AC will be discussed with doctor before dilatation.

Structure

The following resources are required:

- Adequate knowledge and skill to perform assessment of the anterior chamber (learner to be supervised by competent practitioner)
- Pen torch with bright light
- Patient medical records.

Process

The HCP should complete the following steps:

Introduce yourself to the patient, check the identity of the patient and explain the procedure.

To ensure the patient is correctly identified against the medical records and promote the patient's understanding in order to gain cooperation, obtain consent and allay anxiety.

In dim light, ask patient to look straight ahead.

To ensure AC viewed correctly.

Shine pen torch light from temporal side (an angle of 90–100° in the horizontal plane).

To illuminate the temporal side of the iris.

Observe the nasal side of the iris carefully and note how much is in shadow.

To identify the depth of the AC.

- The deep AC will be illuminated across the plane compared to the shallow AC which will have significant shadow on the nasal side.
- The shallow AC will have a shadow cast across the nasal iris.

It may be useful to view the AC from the temporal side view noting the depth between the iris and the cornea.

Document shallow AC in patient records and discuss with doctor whether to proceed with dilatation or ask patient to wait for medical assessment first.

To ensure angle closure does not occur without medical supervision.

Outcomes

The patient will:

understand the procedure

cooperate and fix gaze appropriately

have an accurate assessment of the AC depth

be safely prepared for dilatation prior to medical review if appropriate.

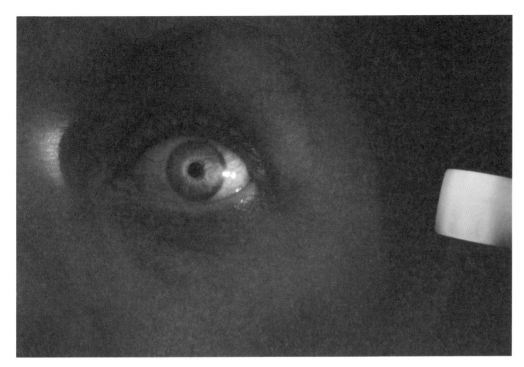

Figure 4 Shadow falling on nasal iris = shallow AC

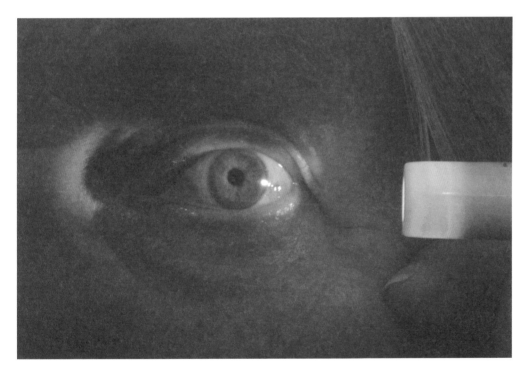

Figure 5 Light seen across iris = deep AC

RELATIVE AFFERENT PUPILLARY DEFECT

All patients will have this test performed to identify whether the reduction in visual acuity is due to a defect in the visual pathway anterior to the optic chiasm, indicating an optic nerve or macular disorder.

Structure

The following resources are required:
- Adequate knowledge and skill to perform assessment of the pupillary function (learner to be supervised by competent practitioner)
- Dimly lit room
- Bright light – ophthalmoscope or bright pen torch
- Patient's medical records.

Process

The HCP should complete the following steps:

Introduce yourself to the patient, check the identity of the patient and explain the procedure.
To ensure the patient is correctly identified against the medical records and promote the patient's understanding in order to gain cooperation, obtain consent and allay anxiety.

Position the patient comfortably in the chair with access to lighting that can be dimmed accordingly.
To aid cooperation and to maximise pupil size therefore accentuating response.

Ask the patient to fix gaze either to a distant object or to your nose if vision is significantly impaired.
Near reflex associated with accommodation and convergence causes the pupils to constrict therefore gaze fixed in the distance is preferable.

Using a very bright light assess direct and consensual pupil response in both eyes.
Absence of a consensual response indicates an abnormality.

Swing very bright light from pupil to pupil approaching temporally for approximately 3 seconds duration. Repeat as necessary to indicate abnormality.
To confirm normal or abnormal results – an eye with a relative afferent pupillary defect will not constrict or will have a sluggish constriction response.

If in any doubt, check with an experienced ophthalmic nurse or medical colleague.
To ensure accuracy when in doubt.

Document outcome in the patient's medical records as follows:
RAPD – graded from 0 (No RAPD) to 4 + (Brisk RAPD).
To ensure accurate documentation of test and provide record of care.
Note: An RAPD is indicated in an eye, in which on alternate illumination, the pupil dilates or has no constrict response when light is directed on the affected eye.
The result can be profound and brisk or subtle and sluggish.

Outcomes

The patient will:

understand and consent to process

be comfortable and able to maintain position during the procedure

gaze in correct position to carry out procedure

have any consensual defect identified.

AMSLER GRID TEST

Standard Statement

All patients with suspected macular disease (when best corrected VA reduced, acquired colour vision anomaly or when central vision distortion is noted) will have an accurate assessment using the Amsler Grid test.

Structure

The following resources are required:

- Adequate knowledge and skill to perform Amsler Grid assessment (learner to be supervised by competent practitioner)
- Amsler Grid sheet
- Occluder
- Adequate illumination source.

Process

The HCP should complete the following steps:

Introduce yourself to the patient, check the identity of the patient and explain the procedure.
To ensure the patient is correctly identified against the medical records and promote the patient's understanding in order to gain cooperation, obtain consent and allay anxiety.

Position the patient comfortably holding the Amsler Grid sheet at reading vision distance.
To maintain correct position and to ensure comfort throughout the procedure.

Ensure good lighting of the chart and the environment.
To ensure optimal and accurate recording of visual acuity.

Establish whether the patient needs refractive correction for near vision and correct where necessary, e.g. ask the patient to wear his/her reading spectacles. The use of refractive aids must be noted in the patient's record.
To ensure that the patient's optimal vision is recorded.

Ask the patient to occlude the affected eye (or worst affected eye).
This will aid cooperation with test and improve understanding and reliability of results.

Ask the patient to look at the central dot without moving the eyes. Are all the lines straight, wavy, any missing? Are all the squares the same size, larger/smaller? Note each response on the sheet.
Identifies normal or least abnormal vision.

Change the occluder to the worst affected eye and repeat.
Identifies any abnormality, distortion etc.

Ensure you observe the patient to ensure fellow eye remains occluded.
Accurate information is obtained.

Ensure the Amsler sheet is accurately marked Right Eye/Left Eye appropriately and securely attached in the patient's medical records

To ensure accurate documentation of test and provide record of care.

Outcomes

The patient will:

understand and consent to procedure

be comfortable and able to maintain position during the procedure

have any defect identified

have an accurate record maintained in their record

SCHIRMER'S TEAR TEST

Standard Statement

Each patient will have an accurate assessment of the quantity of tears produced using the Schirmer's tear test, No.1 (measuring basal and reflex secretion) or No. 2 (with topical anaesthesia – measuring basal tear secretion).

Structure

The following resources are required:

- Adequate knowledge and skill to perform Shirmer's tear test
  (learner to be supervised by competent practitioner)
- Schirmer's tear test filter strips (one for each eye)
- Patient's medical records
- Box of tissues.

Process

The HCP should complete the following steps:

Introduce yourself to the patient, check the identity of the patient and explain the procedure including the discomfort involved.

To ensure the patient is correctly identified against the medical records and promote the patient's understanding in order to gain cooperation, obtain consent and allay anxiety.

Position the patient comfortably in a chair with his/her head well supported.

To maintain correct posture to ensure comfort and reduce movement of the head.

Wash and dry hands thoroughly complying with local infection control guidelines.

To reduce risk of cross contamination with microorganisms.

Both eyes are tested together in a dimly lit room.

To ensure patient's normal tear function is tested and no excess tearing occurs due to photophobia.

Schirmer's 1

Insert top end of folded tear test strips into inferior fornix temporally.

To reduce the risk of corneal abrasion.

Ask the patient to look up or gently close eyes.

To ensure corneal surface is protected, reduce abnormal tearing due to tear stimulation and facilitate comfort.

Leave strips in place for 5 minutes and stay with patient during procedure.

To comply with test requirements for accurate assessment of quantity of tears and provide psychological support during the procedure.

Remove the test strips and measure the dampened area in millimetres (usually there is a gauge provided).

To measure the tear quantity against the accepted standard.

Document procedure and findings in patient's medical records.

To communicate actions and findings to other members of healthcare team.

Results will indicate the following:

- Normal which is > 15mm wetting of the paper after 5 minutes.
- Borderline which is 6–10mm wetting of the paper after 5 minutes
- Impaired which is < 6mm wetting of the paper after 5 minutes.

Dispose of clinical waste according to local infection control guidelines.

To comply with policies and procedures of the organisation.

Wash and dry hands thoroughly complying with local infection control guidelines.

To reduce risk of cross contamination with microorganisms.

Schirmer's 2

Instil one drop of topical local anaesthetic according to local guidelines before carrying out the above steps.

To facilitate basal tear secretion measurement and to provide comfort if procedure not tolerated.

Document Schirmer's 2 in the patient's medical record with the results of the test.

To inform members of the healthcare team that local anaesthetic was used prior to the test and that results may be slightly less than if topical anaesthetic had not been used.

Outcomes

The patient will:

understand and consent to the procedure

be able to cooperate during the procedure

not be exposed to the risk of cross infection

have an accurate measurement of tear function.

Note: Schirmer's 3 can also be tested when the nasal mucosa is irritated with cotton bud tip to provoke reflex tearing (Marsden, J. 2007) but this is not considered within this standard as it is not normal practice within our department.

NASOLACRIMAL SYRINGING

Standard Statement

All patients undergoing syringing of their lacrimal drainage system to assess the patency will go through the procedure safely.

Structure

The following resources are required:

- Adequate knowledge and skill to perform nasolacrimal syringing (learner to be supervised by competent practitioner)
- Clean trolley
- Sterile dressing pack
- Single use lacrimal syringing set which includes: Nettleship dilator if used within own department, and Punctum seeker
- 26g Lacrimal cannula or similar according to local policy
- Normal saline
- 2ml syringe
- Prescribed drugs: Local anaesthetic drops as per local protocol
- Patient's records
- Good lighting
- Access to adequate hand washing facilities.

Process

The HCP should complete the following steps:

Introduce yourself to the patient, check the identity of the patient and explain the procedure.

To ensure the patient is correctly identified against the medical records and promote the patient's understanding in order to gain cooperation, obtain consent and allay anxiety.

Position the patient comfortably in a chair with his/her head well supported and tilted slightly backwards.

To maintain correct posture to ensure comfort and reduce movement of the head.

Wash and dry hands thoroughly complying with local infection control guidelines.

To reduce risk of cross contamination with microorganisms.

Checking against patient's medical records and prescription, instil local anaesthetic drops directly over the punctum to be syringed, following standard of care for instilling drops.

To anaesthetise punctual area prior to syringing. Allow about three minutes for the local anaesthetic to take effect.

Position paper towel appropriately.

To prevent patient's clothing getting wet.

Ask patient to adopt an upward gaze throughout the procedure.
To protect the cornea from accidental injury.

Ascertain punctual patency prior to syringing.
Watering may be caused by malposition, inflammation, stenosis of the puncta or canaliculitis.

Please note that this next step is subject to local policy
Insert the Nettleship (named after Mr Nettleship of St Thomas's Hospital) dilator into patient's lower punctum and follow the passage of the canaliculus, rotating gently en route. (Review anatomy and physiology of lacrimal duct if in any doubt of correct positioning of dilator.)
To dilate the lower punctum and passage to allow insertion of the lacrimal cannula.

Inform patient that he/she may taste salty liquid in the throat and that it may be swallowed. Insert a gently curved 26g blunt tipped lacrimal cannula attached to a 2ml saline-filled syringe into the dilated lower punctum and advance following the contour of the canaliculus and inject the saline slowly
To introduce the fluid into the nasolacrimal passage to ascertain the patency of the system.

Result:

If the patient can feel saline in his nasopharynx and no regurgitation is observed then the lacrimal drainage system is freely patent.

If the patient has reflux through the lower punctum then the obstruction is in the lower canaliculus.

Reflux through the upper punctum indicates patency of both upper and lower canaliculi but obstruction of the common canaliculus or total obstruction which will cause the lacrimal sac to become distended.

Occlude the upper punctum with Nettleship dilator and re-syringe lower punctum.
To ascertain the position of the obstruction.

Document procedure and findings in patient's medical records.
To communicate actions and findings to other members of care team.

Dispose of non-reusable equipment in clinical waste. Place any reusable equipment (if used) for cleaning and sterilisation according to local infection control policy.
To ensure all equipment is re-sterilised in preparation for further use. Note: Always use single use equipment if available

Outcomes

The patient will:

understand and consent to procedure

be comfortable and able to maintain position during the procedure

not be exposed to risk of cross infection.

have any blockage within the lacrimal drainage system identified.

Following further consultation with medical team patient will have sufficient knowledge about
condition to be discharged home.

All reusable equipment to be sterilised and ready for use.

BANDAGE CONTACT LENS INSERTION

Standard Statement

All patients will have their bandage contact lens inserted safely.

Structure

The following resources are required:

- Adequate knowledge and skill to carry out insertion of bandage contact lens (learner to be supervised by competent practitioner)
- Bandage contact lens
- Eye dressing pack
- Tissues
- Access to adequate hand washing facilities.

Process

The HCP should complete the following steps:

Introduce yourself to the patient, check the identity of the patient and explain the procedure.

To ensure the patient is correctly identified against the medical records and promote the patient's understanding in order to gain cooperation, obtain consent and allay anxiety.

Ensure patient is positioned comfortably with head well supported.

To promote comfort and reduce head movement during procedure.

Wash and dry hands thoroughly according to local infection control policy.

To reduce the risk of cross contamination with microorganisms.

Place contact lens on the tip of the index finger.

To aid insertion.

Hold the lids apart with the other hand, retracting the lower lid.

To prevent blinking during insertion.

Ask the patient to look down to retract the upper lid.

To prevent blinking during insertion.

Move the contact lens close to the patient's eye, ask the patient to look straight ahead and at the same time gently but firmly apply the lens to the centre of the cornea.

To position the eye correctly and place in the correct position.

When the lens is stable on the surface of the cornea release the lids and ask the patient to blink.

To help centre the lens in correct position.

Check the position of the lens on the slit lamp or with pen torch.

To ensure the lens is sitting correctly on the corneal surface.

Document procedure and findings in patient's medical record.

To communicate actions and findings to other members of care team.

Dispose of clinical waste according to local infection control guidelines.
To comply with policies and procedures of the organisation.

Outcomes

The patient will:

understand and consent to the procedure

be able to cooperate during the procedure

not be exposed to the risk of cross infection

have contact lens inserted and positioned correctly.

BANDAGE CONTACT LENS REMOVAL

Standard Statement

All patients will have their bandage contact lens removed safely.

Structure

The following resources are required:

- Adequate knowledge and skill to carry out removal of bandage contact lens (learner to be supervised by competent practitioner)
- Eye dressing pack
- Tissues
- Access to adequate hand washing facilities.

Process

The HCP should complete the following steps:

Introduce yourself to the patient, check the identity of the patient and explain the procedure.
To ensure the patient is correctly identified against the medical records and promote the patient's understanding in order to gain cooperation, obtain consent and allay anxiety.

Wash and dry hands thoroughly according to local infection control policy.
To reduce the risk of cross contamination with microorganisms.

Direct patient gaze straight ahead.
To ensure contact lens can be adequately exposed.

Place the tips of your index fingers at lid margins (12 & 6 o\c) retracting the lids. (Do not evert the lids or lens edge may slip underneath.)
To correctly position lids.

Gently press the lids against the globe and move the lids towards each other to scissor the lens until one edge pops up from corneal surface.
To prevent damage to the corneal surface.

Continue to move the lids towards each other until lens is removed. Ask patient to close lids and remove exposed lens.
To completely remove lens without causing corneal damage.

Examine lens to ensure complete removal – check edges.
To ensure whole lens is removed.

Document procedure and findings in patient's medical record.
To communicate actions and findings to other members of care team.

Dispose of clinical waste according to local infection control guidelines.
To comply with policies and procedures of the organization.

Outcomes

The patient will:

understand the procedure

be able to cooperate during the procedure

not be exposed to the risk of cross infection

have contact lens removed safely and completely

have accurate information within records to inform others.

OCULAR HYGIENE

Standard Statement

All patients will feel more comfortable after having their lids and surrounding structures cleaned with normal saline.

Structure

The following resources are required:

- Adequate knowledge and skill to carry out ocular hygiene (learner to be supervised by competent practitioner)
- Eye dressing pack
- Clean dressing trolley
- Normal saline sachet
- Tissues
- Access to adequate hand washing facilities.

Process

The HCP should complete the following steps:

Introduce yourself to the patient, check the identity of the patient and explain the procedure.

To ensure the patient is correctly identified against the medical records and promote the patient's understanding in order to gain cooperation, obtain consent and allay anxiety.

Ask the patient to sit comfortably in a chair with neck supported.

To enable patient to cooperate fully with procedure.

Open pack onto prepared clean surface and wash hands before procedure according to local infection control policy.

To prevent potential cross infection with microorganisms.

Remove any dressing if necessary and again wash hands after removing dressing.

To access site and prevent cross infection with microorganisms.

Fold swabs to ensure hands have not touched edge touching eye.

To prevent cross infection.

Ask patient to close eye and gently clean using one swab to wipe from nasal edge outwards. Repeat as necessary to remove secretions/debris using a clean swab for each wipe.

To avoid corneal damage during procedure and clean lashes of debris which can potentially cause infection.

Ask patient to look up towards the ceiling and lower lid margin gently. Clean whilst holding the lid down, using one swab to wipe from nasal edge outwards. Repeated as necessary using a clean swab for each wipe.

To avoid corneal damage during procedure and clean lashes of debris which can potentially cause infection.

Ask patient to look downwards to remove risk of corneal damage and line of sight.

Upper lid margin gently cleaned by elevating lid away from the globe, using one swab to wipe from the nasal edge outwards. Repeated as necessary using a clean swab for each wipe.

To avoid corneal damage during procedure and clean lashes of debris which can potentially cause infection.

Document ocular hygiene performed and any abnormalities observed in patient's notes.

To ensure accurate recording in patients notes.

Outcomes

The patient will:

understand the procedure

be able to cooperate during the procedure

not be exposed to the risk of cross infection

will have each eye cleaned safely and feel more comfortable following the procedure.

FUNDUS FLUORESCEIN ANGIOGRAPHY

Standard Statement

All patients undergoing a fundus fluorescein angiogram will go through the procedure safely using appropriate interventions without foreseeable adverse reactions and have accurate, timely documentation to support the practice.

All patients will have sufficient, understandable and accurate information in a format that meets their needs to enable them to make an informed decision about the procedure.

Structure

The following resources are required:

- Adequate knowledge and skill to perform FFA (learner to be supervised by competent practitioner)
- Visual acuity equipment – Snellen board, Sheridan–Gardiner, Kay or E cube test
- Access to adequate hand washing facilities
- Accurate, understandable and readable patient information
- Medical photographer and photographic equipment
- Up to date resuscitation equipment
- Doctors present in unit to support emergencies
- Cannulation equipment
- Vital sign monitoring equipment
- Medications
    - IV Fluorescein – 20% conc.
    - Tropicamide 1% eye drops
    - Phenylephrine 2.5% eye drops
- Emergency medications
    - Prochlorperazine IV
    - Piriton, oral & IM/IV
    - Adrenaline/Hydrocortisone IV
    - Emergency cardiac arrest drugs
- All appropriate documentation
    - Medical history assessment
    - FFA care plan
    - Discharge information

Process

The HCP should complete the following steps:

Introduce yourself to the patient, check the identity of the patient and explain the procedure, including how and where it is carried out, about the camera flashes and clicking noises in a relatively dark room.

To ensure the patient is correctly identified against the medical records and promote the patient's understanding in order to gain cooperation, obtain consent and allay anxiety.

Check distance vision using appropriate method according to standard of care.
Identify level of vision before procedure for legal and medical requirements.

Wash and dry hands thoroughly according to local infection control policy.
To reduce the risk of cross contamination with microorganisms.

Check pupils with pen torch according to protocol.
To identify any abnormalities prior to eye drop instillation e.g. relative afferent pupillary defects.

Check patient medical history and understanding of FFA procedure.
To ensure patient gives informed consent and identify any predisposing risk factors for the patient and discuss with medical colleagues.

Check observations of pulse, blood pressure, respirations and visual observation of patient and record.
To obtain baseline observations to assess changes in patient status during procedure.

Explain consent process and ensure patient signs consent form.
To ensure medico-legal requirements are met and patient has given fully informed consent.

Wash and dry hands thoroughly according to local infection control policy.
To reduce the risk of cross contamination with microorganisms.

Cannulate according to local cannulation policy (i.e. 23G Venflon into a big vein in arm and check patency with 5 mls normal saline flush)
To provide IV access to give fluorescein and emergency medication if required.

Check patient details and check prescribed drops.
To ensure that the correct eye drops are given to correct patient.

Explain the effects of the eye drops to the patient.
To ensure patient aware of visual effects of dilating eye drops and to comply with informed consent.

Wash and dry hands thoroughly according to local infection control policy.
To reduce the risk of cross contamination with microorganisms.

Give the prescribed cye drops either prescribed by doctor or under Patient Group Direction.
To dilate pupils of patient prior to procedure.

Wait for approximately 20 minutes and check pupils.
To ensure pupils dilated sufficiently for procedure.

If pupils dilated, proceed with medical photographer to take photos.
To ensure adequate view of retina and retinal vessels.

If not fully dilated, it may be possible to give a further dose of dilating eye drops as above according to local policy and/or agreement with medical colleague.
To ensure pupils dilated sufficiently for procedure.

Give 5 mls 20% fluorescein as prescribed (IV fluorescein is a known unlicensed product but it is not suitable for administration from Patient Group Direction as per NMC (2010), standard 22, section 7) while medical photographer takes photos.

To allow contrast dye to reach retinal vessels quickly to obtain best photos possible.

Observe the patient's colour, respirations, blood pressure and pulse and talk to the patient during the procedure whilst medical photographer takes photos (for approximately 5 mins following fluorescein injection)

To ensure early detection of adverse reactions to fluorescein.

Escort the patient to a safe and comfortable area to relax following procedure. Offer patient a drink.

To ensure able to monitor patient for adverse reactions to fluorescein.

Complete documentation accurately in the patient's medical record.

To provide timely and accurate record of procedure.

Keep a local prospective audit of adverse events for governance reasons and record any adverse event.

To identify all adverse events for audit purposes.

Check patient's BP, P, R and T after 30 minutes.

To ensure early detection of possible adverse reactions.

After 45–60 minutes remove Venflon if patient does not complain of adverse reactions.

To ensure IV access remains available if adverse reactions occur and remove as per local infection control policy.

Give patient advice to support patient information leaflet on signs and symptoms following fluorescein angiography and discharge information before discharging patient home.

To ensure patient able to recognise abnormal reactions following discharge home.

Outcomes

The patient will:

understand what is happening and be able to cooperate with the procedure

have any abnormality or risk factor identified, documented and discussed with medical colleague before procedure

give informed consent for procedure understanding the risks and benefits

have baseline observations documented

have patent IV access

have eye drops given according to protocol and pupils will dilate sufficiently to facilitate good quality photographs to be taken

have IV fluorescein given as per protocol and guidelines

have early detection of adverse symptoms and appropriate action taken

have accurate record of procedure in medical notes and audit of practice facilitated

have observations recorded as returning to normal before discharge

not be discharged with unwanted medical equipment (cannula)

be discharged from hospital with all information needed to self care at home.

Note: NMC guidance on administration of unlicensed products can be found within the NMC (2010) Standards for Medicines Management available at:

http://www.nmc-uk.org/Documents/Standards/nmcStandardsForMedicinesManagementBooklet.pdf (last accessed 23.09.11).

Biometry

Biometry

Background

Biometry is an important aspect of the treatment of various eye conditions using intraocular lenses (IOL). The insertion of intraocular implants dates back to 1949 when Sir Harold Ridley inserted the first artificial lens for pilots who had suffered sight threatening injuries during WWII. Today, the lenses used are either monofocal, for distance vision, or multifocal, which give patients distance and reading (near) vision. Ultrasound biometry or A-scan (echoed sound waves) ultrasound is a diagnostic tool used to determine the eye length pre-operatively for the calculation of the intraocular lens refractive power.

Biometry includes the procedures of measuring the axial length of the eye using A-scan and measuring the power of the cornea (keratometry). The refractive power of an emmetropic eye is approximately 60 diopters; the human cornea provides 40 diopters, and the crystalline lens 20 diopters. Partial Coherence Interferometry (infrared laser) scans the curvature of the cornea (anterior to posterior), anterior chamber depth, the lens thickness and axial length to the retinal pigment epithelium.

Different formulas are used (depending on the features of the individual eye and data collected) to calculate the power of the intraocular lens needed. Today, results from data collection are more accurate and the HCP needs to understand how important accurate data collection is to ensure the correct IOL will be inserted in the correct eye.

The HCP using these types of equipment should familiarise themselves with the manuals supplied with each machine. All eye units/departments will also have different guidelines and policies on infection control and these policies should be adhered to.

Note

For this chapter, IOL Master® by Zeiss (in use since 1999), a non-invasive procedure which most patients find comfortable and E-Z Scan® AB5500+ (contact and immersion scanner) will be discussed as these pieces of equipment are used within the author's work place. It is always recommended that the HCP refers to the manuals available within their own workplace for the specific equipment that they are going to use.

Common abbreviations

OD or Oculus Dexter [Latin] = Right eye
OS or Oculus Sinister [Latin] = Left eye
IOL = Intraocular lens.

BIOMETRY – NON-CONTACT USING IOL MASTER®

All patients will have an accurate biometry documented within the medical records prior to cataract surgery.

Structure

The following resources are required

- Adequate knowledge, skill and competence to perform non-contact biometry using the IOL Master (learner to be supervised by a competent practitioner)
- IOL Master® Biometry machine
- Test Eye instrument
- An office chair, not on castors, that has the function of height adjustment for the patient.
- A similar chair which can be on castors for the HCP
- Access to facilities for hand washing.

Process

The HCP should complete the following *prior to carrying out procedure on any patients.*

Turn machine on and carry out calibration of machine using test eye. This data is to be saved in the main menu screen by selecting NEW.

Each test eye will have a standard measurement or reading that is unique to each eye piece, found printed at the side of the test eye.
To check if machine is working accurately and ensure precision of readings.
The saving of this data can be used for quality assurance purposes.
If at this stage, the data collected from the test eye is inaccurate, switch machine off, refer to manual for troubleshooting or contact the manufacturers' helpdesk for advice.

Introduce yourself to the patient, check the identity of the patient and explain the procedure.
To ensure the patient is correctly identified against the medical records and promote the patient's understanding in order to gain cooperation, obtain consent and reduce potential anxiety.

Open NEW, and enter patient details correctly into the IOL Master®.
To make sure the patient details and measurements will be retained in the machine accurately.

Ensure that no intraocular pressure tonometry or pachymetry has been performed prior to using the IOL Master®
Any contact with the cornea may give a false reading when keratometry is scanned on the IOL Master®.

Ask the patient for a current refractive prescription. If this is unavailable, perform focimetry on current glasses. Note: only measure distance refraction and be particularly careful if multifocal

lenses are worn. Ensure that this measurement is filed within the patient's medical records.

If no current glasses are available, ensure that autorefraction has been carried out. File this in the patient's medical records.

This information will aid the surgeon when choosing the correct IOL for the correct eye.

Ask the patient if there is a history of Laser-Assisted in Situ Keratomileusis (LASIK) or Photorefractive Keratectomy (PRK) surgery.

If the patient confirms that there is a history of a refractive procedure, HCP should refer to own unit/ department standard or policy on refractive surgery before proceeding as K readings will be inaccurate. Topography is a useful tool at this stage. Inform surgeon and document in case notes. If topography has been done, file in patient's medical record.

Position the patient in the chair (no castors) comfortably. The patient should able to rest their chin on chin rest comfortably.

To help patient to cooperate with procedure to take measurement, reduce discomfort and aid compliance.

Position the patient's chin on the chin rest and make sure the patient's eyes are level with line indicator found on either side of the metal frame housing the chin rest. IOL Master® platform can be adjusted for height by using the up and down buttons.

The operating screen can also be adjusted for height for the operator.

To ensure there is access to the visual axis and improve accuracy of measurements taken.

Using the control stick, move the IOL Master® machine to measure the right eye. The screen will indicate (OD) that it has done so. Ask the patient to focus on the red light directly in front with the right eye (OD) onto the light directly in front and (with control stick) place circular guiding display over the pupil seen on the screen.

To ensure machine is in alignment with pupil to improve accuracy of measurements.

Helpful Hint

If patient is unable to focus onto the light directly, carefully occlude fellow eye. This will force the scanned eye to focus on the red light.

Press button on top of control stick for axial length or press A on keyboard. At the bottom of the screen the icon for AL can also be found.

Focus the dots seen on screen to pinpoints. This can be done by moving the control stick backwards or forwards slowly.

To ensure focus correctly.

Ask patient not to blink or move eye whilst measurements are being taken. The HCP should take five measurements of axial length (AL) by clicking the button on top of control stick. The AL images seen will have only one peak. IOL Master® will identify 'error' if lens opacity is too dense for sound waves to penetrate. In this case proceed to contact/immersion biometry.

To acquire an average reading of axial lengths along the visual axis.

Helpful Hints

1. If biometry only is needed for a second eye, it is good practice to take readings for both eyes. Ensure that IOL Master® is moved into position for the eye that has had previous cataract surgery,

using cursor, click on to 'A/L setting', and then click PSEUDOPHAKIC. A second screen will appear with different IOL materials. If the information on the type of IOL used for first eye is documented in the patient's case notes, then click on to selected IOL.

2. For eyes that have had previous retinal surgery with silicone, further down in same screen 'silicone filled eye' should be clicked. The IOL Master® will then reset to take into account the different medium to pass for accurate A/L scans.

3. Where measurements are taken on the A/L screen, the HCP will see the abbreviation 'SNR'. The 'Signal to Noise Ratio' is an evaluation of the scan's accuracy and any reading over 2.0 is an indication of a good scan.

Press button on top of control stick for Keratometry readings or press K on keyboard and focus the circular guidance by moving stick backwards or forwards slowly. Ask patient to blink to improve clarity.

To ensure the image of the eye is focused correctly. Blinking helps to keep eye hydrated – dry eyes have the potential to give inaccurate readings.

Ask the patient to focus on a yellow/orange light. Take three K readings by clicking button on top of control stick. The HCP will see a circle of dots on the screen if the IOL Master® program decides that the readings are incomplete. Delete the highlighted K reading and repeat.

K reading measures the curvature of the cornea and is needed to accurately calculate IOL strength. If keratometry readings are inaccurate, a refractive error or 'surprise' will occur and the implant will have to be removed. Three readings allow for comparison – they should be similar to each other.

Note: If difference is noted between the eyes, check with surgeon. It may not be possible for patients with corneal scarring to get accurate K readings so discuss with the cataract surgeon and document your findings/problems within the patient's medical records. Patients with high astigmatic corneas will have higher K readings – topography may be indicated at this stage.

Using the control stick, position over icon for anterior chamber depth (ACD) or press D on keyboard. Inform patient that a white light will appear. The screen will now change and the HCP will see the image of a rectangle with a dot placed centrally and two white vertical lines. Using the control stick, manoeuver this image centrally on to the pupil ensuring that a vertical line goes through the pupil and the dot is pinpoint. Press once and the IOL Master® will take five readings automatically. The average will be calculated and can be seen as a sixth line.

This information will aid the surgeon when choosing the correct IOL.

Move IOL Master® machine to left eye (OS) and repeat all three steps – AL, K and ACD. Always measure both eyes even if the patient has had cataract surgery in the fellow eye. All measurements should be approximately the same.

To give the surgeon a complete picture of patient with comparative data for both eyes.

Ask patient to sit back in chair but do not allow patient to leave, as readings may need repeating.

To save the patient a repeat attendance to repeat readings.

Check AL, K and ACD readings once more until confident with accuracy of measurements.

To allow for repeat readings if inconsistency appears on recheck. If in doubt, ask a colleague to repeat biometry.

Click button on top of control stick and proceed to IOL calculations section, or choose icon which can be found at the bottom of the screen if cursor is moved into position. If using keyboard, press I.

The HCP should choose the pre-programmed A Constants (where the lens will be positioned in the eye) or IOL calculations from these formulae and following own unit/department guidelines.

Holliday	Hoffer Q	Haggis	SRK T	SRK II

Press IOL print for each formula when calculations appear. If using keyboard, press P.

To give the surgeon a choice of formula to match with AL readings according to Royal College of Ophthalmologist guidelines or print data according to local guidelines.

Check measurements for accuracy – name, date of birth, case number and the correct eye has the correct scanning details. Place printed biometry measurements and calculation into the patient's medical notes and escort patient to the appropriate surgeon.

To ensure correct measurements are in correct patient's notes and available for consultation with surgeon. If the HCP feels the readings are doubtful, ask another HCP to check and if necessary repeat. Ensure the operating surgeon is aware and document in notes.

Inform surgeon biometry completed and patient waiting for consultation.

To improve communication between professionals and patient.

When not in use, turn machine off, go to 'door' icon at bottom right of main menu. Using cursor on keyboard left hand click onto icon. Select 'ok' for lockdown. The machine will then indicate to switch off.

Wash and dry hands thoroughly.

The HCP should follow own organisation's infection control policy on hand washing to reduce the risk of cross infection.

Outcomes

The patient will:

understand and consent to having biometry

understand the risks and benefits

have correct eye(s) scanned with the correct biometry readings documented in the medical records.

Note: There are a number of versions ranging from V1 to V5 for the IOL Master® so you must be aware which IOL Master® software version you are using within your own workplace. They generally are used in a similar fashion but you may need to carry out various other functions on more up-to-date models e.g. 'white on white' measurements.

BIOMETRY –
CONTACT USING E-Z Scan® AB5500+

Standard Statement

All patients will have an accurate biometry documented within the medical records prior to cataract surgery.

Structure

The following resources are required

- Adequate knowledge, skill and competence to perform contact biometry using the E-Z Scan (learner to be supervised by a competent practitioner)
- E-Z Scan® AB5500 +
- Test Eye piece for E-Z Scan® AB5500 +
- Ultrasound gel as recommended by E-Z Scan® AB5500 + (manufacturers')
- Local anaesthetic drops within expiry date
- A reclining chair, not on castors, that has the function of height adjustment for the patient
- An office chair which can be on castors for the HCP
- Tissues
- Access to facilities for hand washing.

Process

The HCP should complete the following steps *prior to carrying out procedure on any patients.*

1. Switch on scanner (found at the back) and printer. Ensure that foot pedal is placed within reach on the floor.
2. Scanner screen will light up and show menu with options to choose. This is a touch screen, select 'A scan' using control pen.
3. Apply a small amount of ultrasound gel to eye piece (small round clear plastic) found on right side of scanner.
4. This piece will have a number attached which will have a reading of 10mm ± 0.1 which is the preferred correct calibration for this machine. This is the indicated pass test for this machine. Press foot pedal once.
5. Using probe device (this can be found when not in use in designated holder), press on to test piece as flat as possible. The HCP should continue until a frozen image appears.
6. Calibration is now confirmed. Print reading and file.
7. Clean probe and test piece.

To check if machine is working accurately and ensure precision of readings. The saving of this data can be used for quality control. If at this stage, the data collected from the test eye is inaccurate, switch machine off, refer to manual or to the manufacturers' helpdesk for advice.

Introduce yourself to the patient, check the identity of the patient and explain the procedure when the patient arrives.

To ensure the patient is correctly identified against the medical records and promote the patient's understanding in order to gain cooperation, obtain consent and allay anxiety.

The HCP can now enter patient details by using control pen. Click on 'USER 1:' The screen will change, using control pen pick 'patient' then 'new patient'. The image of a keyboard will now appear on the screen. Following the screen format, enter name, surname, unique patient number and eye to be scanned, pressing 'enter' at all stages. Now click 'Done' and the screen will change to A SCAN display screen.

To make sure the patient details and measurements will be retained in the machine accurately. Note: this scanner will only retain the last patient's details as opposed to IOL Master® which can store many.

The HCP should be able to see on the A Scan display screen at the top right:
1. Patient's details.
2. Which eye to be scanned – indicated as OD or OS.
3. 5 lines for scanning details – blank.
4. ACD – blank.
5. Lens thickness – blank.
6. Average AL – blank.

If at this stage, the data shown is incorrect, do not proceed further. Refer to manual for troubleshooting or contact the manufacturers' helpdesk for advice.

Wash and dry hands thoroughly.

The HCP should follow own organisation's infection control policy on hand washing to reduce the risk of cross infection.

Check with patient and their medical records for known allergies to medications and eye drops. Document any findings in patient's medical records.

To reduce risk of adverse reactions and promote communication between patient and the healthcare professional.

Explain procedure to patient gaining consent.

To gain consent and cooperation for procedure, and ensure understanding.

Ensure patient is positioned comfortably with head well supported.

To ensure comfort and reduce movement of head during procedure.

Wash and dry hands thoroughly.

The healthcare professional should follow own organisation's infection control policy on hand washing to reduce the risk of cross infection.

Instil one drop of local anaesthetic into the lower fornix without touching the eye, the lids or lashes.

For the unregistered HCP, ensure you follow local guidelines which may include obtaining a countersignature for administration of eye drop POM. Only one drop will be held in the eye, as additional drops will spill over the lid margins. Non-contact drop instillation will prevent cross infection. Anaesthetic is necessary to ensure compliance as this procedure is uncomfortable.

Ask patient to relax neck and gently close the eye avoiding the tendency to squeeze the eye closed.

This will allow time for absorption of drops.

The patient can gently wipe away any excess drops with the clean tissue if able. Dispose of the tissue for the patient in the nearest clinical waste bin.

For the patient's comfort and to prevent possible skin irritation. To prevent cross infection.

Ensure that the patient is sitting comfortably and can look up without discomfort. Select 'Measure' on scanner.

To ensure comfort and reduce movement of head during procedure.

Before performing an axial length measurement, using control pen, enter cataract, dense cataract, aphakic, or pseudophakic on touch screen (found top right hand of screen). The E-Z Scan® AB5500 + scanner needs this information for A-Scan calculations and to avoid refractive surprises.

Press foot pedal once.

The HCP should hold probe in dominant hand.

1. Ask patient to focus straight ahead (red light at tip of probe) as the probe needs to align on the patient's visual axis for accurate scans.
2. The Gain control (right side of scanner) can be used to increase the strength or decibel of the echo.
3. Use probe to gently touch cornea. Automatic scanning with peaks will commence.
4. If the scans are acceptable to the A/L program, an image of a frozen scan will appear accompanied by high pitched noise.
5. The HCP should press the foot pedal once if the scan is acceptable. The frozen scan indicated will be seen in top centre of screen marked 'SCAN 1'. Five scans should be entered for best comparison.
6. All scans should have five spikes to right of image, large gap and a defined first spike to left of image. Any other spikes seen after defined spike will be orbital fat.
7. Review when completed. Print scan, ensuring that the scan has either OR or OS indicated.
8. To discard any scans click on 'DEL SCAN'. To delete all scans click on 'CLR ALL'.
9. Print scan and secure within the patient's medical records.

Using control pen, touch screen to change to fellow eye.

Explain procedure to patient gaining consent.

To gain consent and cooperation for procedure, and to ensure understanding.

Ensure patient is positioned comfortably with head well supported.

To ensure comfort and reduce movement of head during procedure.

Instil one drop of local anaesthetic into the lower fornix without touching the eye, the lids or lashes.

For the unregistered HCP, ensure you follow local guidelines which may include obtaining a countersignature for administration of eye drop POM. Only one drop will be held in the eye, as additional drops will spill over the lid margins. Non-contact drop instillation will prevent cross infection. This procedure for contact biometry is uncomfortable as the corneal surface is touched by the probe and to ensure compliance anaestetic is necessary.

Ask patient to relax neck and gently close the eye avoiding the tendency to squeeze the eye closed.

This will allow time for absorption of drops.

The patient can gently wipe away any excess drops with the clean tissue if able. Dispose of the tissue for the patient in the nearest clinical waste bin.

For the patient's comfort and to prevent possible skin irritation. To prevent cross infection.

For second eye (if needed) the HCP must ensure that a scan of first eye has been printed.

To make sure patient details and correct measurements for the correct eye are retained in the machine.

Using control pen, touch screen to change to fellow eye.

The HCP should repeat the steps as for the first eye.

Check measurements for accuracy – name, date of birth, case number and that the correct eye has the correct scanning details.

Place printed scan measurements into the patient's medical notes.

To allow surgeon access to these measurements and ensure that the measurements that have been entered into the IOL Master® are accurate.

The HCP needs to add these measurements to the IOL Master® according to local policy and guidelines.

The HCP should choose the pre-programmed A Constants (where the lens will be positioned in the eye) or IOL calculations from these formulae following own unit/department guidelines.

Holliday	Hoffer Q	Haggis	SRK T	SRK II

Press IOL print for each formula when calculations appear. If using keyboard, press P.

To give the surgeon choice of formula to match with AL readings according to Royal College of Ophthalmologist guidelines or print according to local policy and guidelines.

Check measurements for accuracy – name, date of birth, case number and that the correct eye has the correct scanning details. Place printed biometry measurements and calculation into the patient's medical records and escort patient to the appropriate surgeon.

To ensure correct measurements are in correct patient's notes and available for consultation with surgeon. If the HCP feels the readings are doubtful, ask another HCP to check and if necessary repeat. Ensure the operating surgeon is aware and document in notes.

Inform surgeon biometry completed and patient waiting for consultation.

To improve communication between professionals and patient.

Wash and dry hands thoroughly.

The HCP should follow own organisation's infection control policy on hand washing to reduce the risk of cross infection.

Outcomes

The patient will:

understand and consent to having biometry

understand the risks and benefits

have correct eye(s) scanned with the correct biometry readings documented in the medical records.

Note: There are many contact biometry machines available within the marketplace and you should ensure you follow the guidelines outlined in the manual for the specific equipment available within your own workplace.

You may choose to make a standard similar to this one for your own specific equipment for use within your workplace.

BIOMETRY – IMMERSION

Standard Statement

All patients will have an accurate biometry documented within the medical records prior to cataract surgery.

Structure

The following resources are required

- Adequate knowledge, skill and competence to perform immersion biometry using E-Z Scan (learner to be supervised by a competent practitioner)
- E-Z Scan® AB5500+
- Test Eye piece for E-Z Scan® AB5500+
- Prager immersion shell
- Ultrasound gel as recommended by E-Z Scan® AB5500+ (manufacturers')
- Ampoules of 5mls of normal saline
- 5ml syringe
- 14 NON-DEHP MINIBORE extension set (single use only) which should be sealed and within expiry date
- Sterile water
- Local anaesthetic drops within expiry date
- A reclining chair, not on castors that has the function of height adjustment for the patient
- Tissues
- Clean towel
- Access to facilities for hand washing.

Process

The HCP should complete the following *prior to carrying out procedure on any patients.*

1. Switch on scanner (found at the back) and printer. Ensure that foot pedal is placed within reach on the floor.
2. Scanner screen will light up and show menu with options to choose. This is a touch screen. Select 'A scan' using pen device.
3. Apply a small amount of ultrasound gel to eye piece (small round clear plastic) found on right side of scanner.
4. This piece will have a number attached which will have a reading of 10mm ± 0.1 which is the preferred correct calibration for this machine. This is the indicated pass test for this machine. Press foot pedal once.
5. Using probe device (this can be found when not in use in designated holder), press on to test piece as flat as possible. The HCP should continue until a frozen image appears. Calibration is now confirmed.
6. Print reading and file.
7. Clean probe and test piece.

To check if machine is working accurately and ensure precision of readings. The saving of this data can be used for quality control. If at this stage, the data collected from the test eye is inaccurate, switch machine off, refer to manual or to the manufacturer's helpdesk for advice.

➡ Helpful hint

It is good practice at the beginning of clinic to soak/immerse the Prager shell(s) in the sterilising solution as per manufacturer's recommendation. At the end of clinic day, discard this solution safely.

Introduce yourself to the patient, check the identity of the patient and explain the procedure when patient arrives.

To ensure the patient is correctly identified against the medical records and promote the patient's understanding in order to gain cooperation, obtain consent and allay anxiety.

The HCP can now enter patient details by using control pen. Click on 'USER 1:' The screen will change, using control pen pick 'patient' then 'new patient'. The image of a keyboard will now appear on the screen.

Following the screen format, enter name, surname, unique patient number and eye to be scanned pressing 'enter' at all stages. Now click 'Done' and the screen will change to A SCAN display screen.

To make sure the patient details and measurements will be retained in the machine accurately.

Note: this scanner will only retain the last patient's details as opposed to IOL Master® which can store many.

The HCP should be able to see on the A Scan display screen at the top right

1. Patient's details.

2. Which eye to be scanned – indicated as OD or OS.

3. 5 lines for scanning details – blank.

4. ACD – blank.

5. Lens thickness – blank.

6. Average AL – blank.

If at this stage, the data shown is incorrect, do not proceed further. Refer to manual for troubleshooting or contact the manufacturers' helpdesk for advice.

Check with patient and notes for known allergies to medications and eye drops. Document any findings in patient's notes.

To reduce risk of adverse reactions and promote communication between patient and the healthcare professional.

Explain procedure to patient, gaining consent.

To gain consent and cooperation for procedure, and to ensure understanding.

Using control pen, immersion program needs to be turned on by clicking 'IMMER' seen on the screen. Ensure patient is positioned comfortably with head well supported.

To ensure comfort and reduce movement of head during procedure.

Wash and dry hands thoroughly.

The healthcare professional should follow own organisation's infection control policy on hand washing to reduce the risk of cross infection.

Instil one drop of local anaesthetic into the lower fornix without touching the eye, the lids or lashes. Place a clean paper towel over the patient's shoulder to keep clothing dry.

For the unregistered HCP, ensure you follow local guidelines which may include obtaining a countersignature for administration of eye drop POM. Only one drop will be held in the eye, as additional drops will spill over the lid margins. Non-contact drop instillation will prevent cross infection. This procedure is uncomfortable and to ensure compliance anaesthetic is necessary.

Ask patient to relax neck and gently close the eye avoiding the tendency to squeeze the eye closed.
This will allow time for absorption of drops.

The patient can gently wipe away any excess drops with the clean tissue if able. Dispose of the tissue for the patient in the nearest clinical waste bin.
For the patient's comfort and to prevent possible skin irritation. To prevent cross infection

Ensure that the Prager shell is rinsed with sterile water and dry thoroughly.
The sterilising solution will be harmful to the patient's eye. Sterilising will prevent cross infection.

Wash and dry hands thoroughly.
The HCP should follow own organisation's infection control policy on hand washing to reduce the risk of cross infection.

The HCP now needs to:
1. Unscrew the probe and carefully insert the probe tip on to the Prager shell.
2. The tip has to be parallel with the line found notched in the Prager shell.
3. When in position, to hold the probe in place, tighten the white nylon screw.
4. Attach 14 NON-DEHP MINIBORE extension set.
5. Fill the 5 ml syringe with 5 mls of normal saline.
6. Attach syringe to 14 NON-DEHP MINIBORE extension set.

This will ensure that accurate measurements can be taken.

The HCP should rest the syringe on the towel placed on the patient's shoulder.
1. Hold on to the shell with probe.
2. Elevate the upper lid and insert the flared rim of the Prager shell gently underneath the lid.
3. When in place, ask the patient to look straight ahead toward the red fixation light in the probe tip.
4. Pull the patient's lower lid down and gently insert the lower rim of the shell into the lower fornix taking care not to touch the cornea.
5. Press the foot pedal once.
6. Pick up the syringe from the patient's shoulder and begin to slowly inject the normal saline into the shell.
7. When the injected normal saline reaches the tip of the probe (approximately 2mls), the waveforms of immersion biometry will be seen on screen.

If the scans are acceptable to the immersion program, an image of a frozen scan will appear accompanied by a high pitched noise.

The HCP should press the foot pedal once if the scan is acceptable. This will be seen in top centre of screen marked 'SCAN 1. Five scans will automatically be entered, check for best comparison.

All scans should have five spikes to right of image, large gap and a defined first (retinal) spike to left of image. Any other spikes seen after defined spike will be orbital fat. The ACD and lens thickness will also be indicated.

Review when completed. Print scan, ensuring that the scan has either OR or OS indicated.

To discard any scans click 'DEL SCAN'. To delete all scans click 'CLR ALL'.

1. Check the scans for accuracy.
2. Holding the shell in a downward position, remove the Prager shell ensuring you do not touch the cornea.
3. Any solution left in the Prager shell should then fall on to the patient's cheek. Offer a clean tissue to wipe the excess away. Dispose of this in the nearest clinical waste bin.

For the patient's comfort and to prevent possible skin irritation. To prevent cross infection.

For second eye (if needed), the HCP professional must ensure that a printed scan of first eye has been printed.

To make sure the patient details and the correct measurements for the correct eye will be retained in the machine accurately.

Using control pen, touch screen to change to fellow eye.

The HCP should repeat the steps for the first eye.

Check measurements for accuracy – name, date of birth, case number and the correct eye has the correct scanning details.

Place printed scan measurements into the patient's medical notes.

The HCP needs to add these measurements to the IOL Master®.

The HCP should choose the pre-programmed A Constants (where the lens will be positioned in the eye) or IOL calculations from these formulae following own unit/department guidelines.

Holliday	Hoffer Q	Haggis	SRK T	SRK II

Press IOL print for each formula when calculations appear. If using keyboard, press P.

To give the surgeon a choice of formula to match with AL readings according to Royal College of Ophthalmologist guideline or print according to local policy and guidelines.

Check measurements for accuracy – name, date of birth, case number and that the correct eye has the correct scanning details. Place printed biometry measurements and calculations into the patient's medical notes and escort patient to the appropriate surgeon.

To ensure correct measurements are in correct patient's notes and available for consultation with surgeon. If the HCP feels the readings are doubtful, ask another HCP to check and if necessary repeat. Ensure the operating surgeon is aware and document in notes.

Discard used single use 14 NON-DEHP MINIBORE extension set and syringe as per local policy on waste disposal.

Inform surgeon biometry completed and patient waiting for consultation.

To improve communication between professionals and patient.

Wash and dry hands thoroughly

The HCP should follow own organisation's infection control policy on hand washing to reduce the risk of cross infection

Outcomes

The patient will:

> understand and consent to having biometry

> understand the risks and benefits

> have correct eye(s) scanned with the correct biometry readings documented within the medical record.

Note: There are many immersion biometry machines available within the marketplace and you should ensure you follow the guidelines outlined in the manual for the specific equipment available within your own workplace.

You may choose to make a standard similar to this one for your own specific equipment for use within your workplace.

The Ophthalmic Accident and Emergency Department

The Ophthalmic Accident and Emergency Department

The nurse working in the A&E department will use all the skills that she has learnt within the outpatient department such as Schirmer's test and use of bandage lenses as well as beginning to develop new competences to meet the needs of ophthalmic emergency patients. The ophthalmic A&E nurse needs to develop new ways of thinking to meet these new challenges.

The major role will be to quickly ascertain the priority given to the patient even though all patients arriving in the A&E department will be concerned about their condition.

In every A&E department the nurse will carry out clinical decision making processes informed by their history taking. New arrivals do not plan their appearance in the department so a system of prioritisation or triage must take place. Shaw *et al.* (2010) highlight the need for the nurse working in the A&E dept to understand the nature of ophthalmic emergencies and be aware of emergency conditions. However the new nurse to an ophthalmic A&E department may not be aware of the signs and symptoms associated with ophthalmic emergency conditions so it is important to have a triage system in place. Field and Tillotson (2008) suggest that initial contact with the patient requires the nurse to summarise relevant information and decide on the correct clinical pathway for the patient's presenting condition. This will require the nurse to be accurate during history taking.

History taking in A&E must include specific reference to a range of information such as when, where, what, how and why events and complaints arise, as emergency conditions may not always be easily identifiable.

An example: Patient   *'Something went in my eye yesterday at work'*

Initial impression   *Foreign body in right eye.*

Additional information   *Foreign body entered right eye when working with ammonia substance which solidifies when exposed to air. No immediate irrigation by patient. Pain score: 6. Red eye.*

The information about the substance that went into the eye should initiate immediate irrigation to remove the chemical. If the nurse had not probed the initial explanation given by the patient, serious consequences could have occurred leading to permanent damage to this patient's right eye. This highlights the need to explore information and ask appropriate questions about what went in the eye, what was happening, were they using protective eyewear? These questions would have triggered initial irrigation even before visual acuity was measured.

Triage is an essential skill for all ophthalmic nurses as patients tend not to arrive in a timely fashion (Marsden, 2006). Recognition of what constitutes an ophthalmic emergency requiring immediate attention and the value of enhanced history taking skills should be the first priority for the nurse new to an ophthalmic A&E department.

The nurse will also need to be able to carry out a number of specialist procedures or investigations to support the patient and facilitate timely diagnosis, such as colour vision, RAPD and dilatation, Schirmer's test and Amsler grid testing. However much of the ophthalmic nurse's role in A&E occurs following diagnosis.

Eye padding may be one of the first skills the new nurse will learn but it must be noted that this is no longer the preferred treatment for all patients with a corneal injury. Marsden (2006) explains that padding is a comfort measure rather than an aid to healing. Padding should be considered as a comfort aid to prevent irritation of the damaged corneal epithelium by the eyelid. It appears that the main benefit of padding the eye is to keep the eyelid closed therefore it needs to be applied firmly. Many units now do not routinely apply a pad unless the patient declares increased comfort with the eye closed. It is considered beneficial in some units to leave the pad off patients with corneal injuries to increase adherence to topical treatments. This should be discussed at local level within the multidisciplinary team to decide on a local policy. However it is for the nurse in the ophthalmic unit to ensure the pad is applied for the correct reason and not on historical habits alone.

Some other simple comfort measures undertaken by ophthalmic nurses in the Ophthalmic A&E department include taping of the lower lid, removing corneal irritation from eyelashes in patients with an inversion of the lid margin (entropion) and removal of misdirected eyelashes (trichiasis) often caused by involutional changes and posterior lamellae scarring (superior or inferior), a procedure called epilation.

The ophthalmic nurse may be required to take eye swabs in ophthalmic outpatient clinics or A&E, however it is likely to be more common in A&E particularly when considering swabs for chlamydia. Swabs should always be taken according to local policy but a guide has been included to assist the new nurse in A&E.

The experienced A&E ophthalmic nurse may develop additional skills to identify particular problems and the new nurse should seek opportunities to augment their skills to provide efficient, effective care within the department. Everting the eyelid is important in ocular irrigation and to identify the presence of a sub-tarsal foreign body. This may be suspected if a patient complains that blinking makes the pain or foreign body sensation worse. This is due to the foreign body scratching the upper corneal surface. The nurse will be able to identify the cause of this pain and remove the foreign body if possible.

The ophthalmic nurse's role in the A&E dept is always varied and often demanding. Balancing the needs of the patients, the prioritisation of individuals over those already waiting and performing a variety of procedures makes a day in A&E stimulating and thought-provoking. The ophthalmic nurse should take every opportunity to develop their ophthalmic nursing knowledge, understanding and competence.

HISTORY TAKING IN CLINIC AND CASUALTY

Standard Statement

All patients will have an accurate history taken and documented in clinical notes as an Accident & Emergency attendee resulting in a precise triage.

Structure

The following resources are required:

- Adequate knowledge and skill to obtain an accurate history from the patient (learner to be supervised by competent practitioner)
- Adequate knowledge and skill to link history, signs and symptoms to a prioritisation/triage category
- Patient Medical Notes and/or A&E record
- Private area for assessment.

Process

The HCP should complete the following steps:

Introduce yourself to the patient, check the identity of the patient and explain the procedure.

To ensure the patient is correctly identified against the medical records and promote the patient's understanding in order to gain cooperation, obtain consent and allay anxiety.

Ask patient about present history of condition:

Be precise and ask patient appropriate questions about present condition, symptoms and duration, e.g. if in pain ask about nature of pain, where is pain?, is pain throbbing, aching or sore?

Note: Remember to try to ask what happened, when did it happen?, where did this happen? (what was the patient doing at the time?), how did it happen? (any preceding event e.g. trauma?).

To aid diagnosis, and to proceed with any investigation, e.g. orthoptic assessment, blood test, dilatation of pupils, if needed following discussion with doctor. This would reduce waiting time for the patient and aid the ophthalmologist with diagnosis, thus enabling casualty clinic to proceed smoothly.

Ask about any previous ophthalmic history, e.g. eye operations, family history like glaucoma or genetic problems.

To aid diagnosis that might be related to past history.

Ask about any known family ophthalmic problems such as glaucoma, unexplained blindness.

To identify any known risk factor linked to ophthalmic conditions such as glaucoma. Many ophthalmic conditions have familial traits or genetic predisposition and therefore these patients are more at risk of developing the disease themselves. However remember that family history is not always known and unexplained blindness can highlight unknown risk factors.

Ask about any past or present medical history and medication.

To ascertain if any medical problems or medication that patient is taking is related to an ophthalmic problem, e.g. history of diabetes, hypertension, thyroid disease, CVA and/or TIA, spondylitis, Crohn's or rheumatoid arthritis.

Medications like warfarin, oral steroids and some antidepressants have an ophthalmic effect as well as interact with topical preparations that may be prescribed. Over-the-counter medications such as topical antibiotics should also be checked.

Ask about social factors that may influence structure and function of both the eye and the whole body.

To establish risk factors of known ophthalmic disease such as smoking and macular degeneration, poor liver function in a heavy drinker, frequent attendance at Outpatients affecting employment and driving with poor visual acuity. These facts may influence the development of a suitable plan of care for the individual patient.

Record visual acuity as per standard of care.

To obtain baseline data and comply with legal requirements.

Examine the eye with pen torch in a systematic manner documenting abnormalities if found, checking anterior chamber depth and for relative afferent pupillary defect as per standards of care if dilatation is required.

To aid diagnosis, provide safe nursing interventions and provide the clinician with a complete history.

If necessary perform ocular hygiene as per standard of care.

To provide patient comfort and remove debris from ocular structures facilitating adequate examination.

All information should be documented in the patient's record.

To provide a clear record of nursing intervention and reduce repetition for the patient.

Patient should be asked to wait in the A&E waiting room and A&E records should be placed within the A&E area in accordance with the appropriate triage category. The patient should be informed of any waiting time and be kept informed if this waiting time changes for any reason.

To ensure patient is seen by the correct clinician at the appropriate time or is kept informed of any unexpected delays.

Outcomes

The patient will:

understand what is happening and be able to cooperate with the procedure

not have to repeat information as full ophthalmic history is documented in medical notes

have any abnormality identified, documented and discussed with medical colleague before continuing with other procedures such as dilatation of pupils

be seen according to triage category with appropriate healthcare professional

be kept informed of any delay to A&E patient flow.

EYE PADDING

Standard Statement

All patients will have a secure padding applied to the affected eye and understand why it is vital to the recovery of the affected eye if required (NB padding is not recommended routinely for care of corneal abrasion, however at times eye padding is vital to the recovery of the eye, e.g. retrobulbar injections).

Structure

The following resources are required:

- Adequate knowledge and skill to apply a firm eye pad (learner to be supervised by competent practitioner)
- Sterile eye pads x 2
- Micropore/Transpore tape as appropriate
- Scissors
- Normal saline eye drops
- Patient Medical Notes and/or A&E record.

Process

The HCP should complete the following steps:

Introduce yourself to the patient, check the identity of the patient and explain the procedure.

To ensure the patient is correctly identified against the medical records and promote the patient's understanding in order to gain cooperation, obtain consent and allay anxiety.

Explain why the pad is required to keep the lid closed to improve comfort.

To ensure the patient understands why the pad is required and is able to remove (if local policy dictates) if lid does not remain closed under the pad.

Ask patient to close both eyes. Fold one pad in half and apply to the affected eye. *Figure 6)*

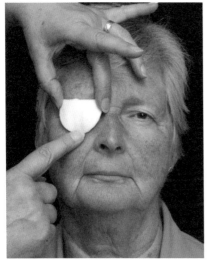 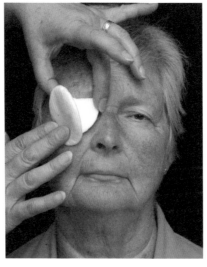 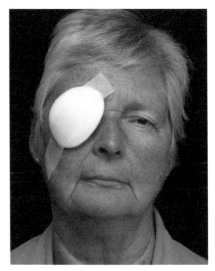

Figure 6 *Figure 7* *Figure 8*

Apply the second pad – unfolded – on top of the first folded pad. *(Figure 7)*

Secure with tape. *(Figure 8)*

To ensure eye is closed for safety and comfort, to promote corneal epithelial healing.

Ask the patient to open his/her eyes and verbally check whether the padded eye has remained shut under the eye pad.

To ensure correct upper lid position maintained when fellow eye is open. If the affected eye has opened below the pad, it is possible to tape the affected upper eyelid in place according to local policy.

Document procedure according to NMC (2010) record keeping guidelines.

To ensure accurate record in patient's medical notes.

Give information about care at home to patient appropriately.

To ensure patient has enough information to be safely self caring at home.

Dispose of non-reusable equipment and waste into a yellow waste bin according to Trust infection control guidelines.

To comply with policies and procedures of the organisation.

Outcomes

The patient will:

understand and consent to procedure

be comfortable and able to maintain position during the procedure

understand how to comply with treatment

not be exposed to risk of cross infection

have a pad applied appropriately and discomfort reduced

have accurate record of treatment in medical notes

be able to self care appropriately.

OCULAR IRRIGATION FOLLOWING CHEMICAL INJURY

Standard Statement

All patients will have thorough irrigation to clean the eye of foreign substances, e.g. multiple foreign bodies and especially corrosive matter such as acid and alkaline burns.

Structure

The following resources are required:

- Adequate knowledge and skill to carry out ocular irrigation (learner to be supervised by competent practitioner)
- Clean trolley
- G. Proxymetacaine or similar local anaesthetic eye drop according to local policy
- Litmus paper
- IV Bag of 0.9% Normal Saline Solution at room temperature and IV giving set
- Receiver
- Cotton buds
- Protection for patient clothing.

Process

The HCP should complete the following steps:

Introduce yourself to the patient, check the identity of the patient and explain the procedure.

To ensure the patient is correctly identified against the medical records and promote the patient's understanding in order to gain cooperation, obtain consent and allay anxiety.

Ensure patient is positioned comfortably reclined with head well supported.

To promote comfort and reduce head movement during procedure.

Wash and dry hands thoroughly

To reduce the risk of cross contamination of microorganisms.

If patient attended A&E following an acute chemical injury, irrigate eye prior to obtaining personal details or VA. Establish basic general health, allergy status and pH only.

To prevent further chemical burn injury by delaying for history and details.

If not acute, obtain personal details and establish pH of the eye.

Delay has already occurred therefore chemical burn established.

Instil local anaesthesia to affected eye. It should be possible to continue to add local anaesthesia as required by the patient as effective irrigation will rapidly leech out this local anaesthetic effect but ensure local guidelines for the use of topical local anaesthetic eye drops are applied in each individual case.

To promote cooperation.

Irrigate eyelids and eye through all extremities of gaze and though upper and lower fornices with a minimum of a litre of sterile saline administered via IV giving set. Note: Evert superior lids to ensure maximum exposure to irrigation fluid.

To prevent any chemicals from remaining within the eye and continuing to burn the ocular surfaces, particularly burning the conjunctiva.

Wait for 10 minutes and assess pH.

To ensure accurate pH obtained and not influenced by irrigation fluid.

If pH 7, assess patient and pass patient through to doctor for ocular assessment.

To ensure normal tear pH is obtained prior to medical assessment.

If pH > 7, continue irrigation until pH returns to 7 then to doctor for assessment.

As above.

Give patient supporting verbal and written information about treatment regimes and arrange follow up visit if required.

To ensure patient understands self care responsibilities and will be followed up appropriately.

Document procedure according to NMC (2010) record keeping guidelines.

To ensure accurate recording in patients notes.

Dispose of non-reusable equipment and waste into a yellow waste bin according to Trust infection control guidelines.

To comply with policies and procedures of the organisation.

Outcomes

The patient will:

understand the procedure

be able to cooperate during the procedure

not be exposed to the risk of cross infection

have all chemicals removed from the ocular structures appropriately

feel as comfortable as possible during the procedure

have accurate post irrigation pH documented in notes

be able to comply with the appropriate treatment regime as prescribed

understand importance of compliance

have accurate record to inform others.

EVERTING EYELIDS

Standard Statement

All patients will undergo lid eversion to facilitate examination of superior palpebral conjunctiva.

Structure

The following resources are required:

- Adequate knowledge and skill to carry out everting lids
  (learner to be supervised by competent practitioner)
- Access to hand washing facilities
- Sterile cotton buds.

Process

The HCP should complete the following steps:

Introduce yourself to the patient, check the identity of the patient and explain the procedure.
To ensure the patient is correctly identified against the medical records and promote the patient's understanding in order to gain cooperation, obtain consent and allay anxiety.

Ensure patient is positioned comfortably with head well supported.
To promote comfort and reduce head movement during procedure.

Wash and dry hands thoroughly.
To reduce the risk of cross contamination of microorganisms.

Ask the patient to look down and grasp the superior eyelashes.
To prevent corneal damage, gain cooperation and facilitate eversion

Press gently on superior margin of tarsal plate using a cotton bud (or index finger of other hand) and at the same time, pull the eyelashes up and out until lid everted.
To facilitate examination of upper palpebral conjunctiva.

During examination, tell patient not to blink and give reassurance all the time lid is everted.
To gain cooperation of patient.

Once examination complete, ask the patient to blink and holding lashes, gently pull away from eye.
To invert lid back to normal position.

To evert lower lid if required:
Pull the lower lid down, pressing under the eyelid margin while moving finger upwards. Lid will evert over the finger. Continue as above.

Outcomes

The patient will:

understand the procedure

be able to cooperate during the procedure

not be exposed to the risk of cross infection

have palpebral conjunctiva examined completely and safely.

CONJUNCTIVAL AND VIRAL SWAB

Standard Statement

Each patient requiring a conjunctival swab to identify any infective organism will be fully informed of the procedure and expectation post procedure.

Structure

The following resources are required:

- Adequate knowledge and skill to take a conjunctival swab
  (learner to be supervised by competent practitioner)
- Appropriate swabs
- Normal saline eye drops or similar to wash away any remaining fluorescein topical dye
- Access to hand washing facilities
- Patient records and swab request card
- Disposable gloves.

Process

The HCP should complete the following steps:

Introduce yourself to the patient, check the identity of the patient and explain the procedure. including likely timeline for results

To ensure the patient is correctly identified against the medical records and promote the patient's understanding in order to gain cooperation, obtain consent and allay anxiety.

Ensure patient is positioned comfortably reclined with head well supported.

To promote comfort and reduce head movement during procedure.

Wash and dry hands thoroughly.

To reduce the risk of cross contamination of microorganisms.

Remove any excess fluorescein topical dye with topical normal saline eyedrops or similar according to local policy.

To remove any potential contaminant from the area to be swabbed.

Open and label swab from packet.

Equipment prepared and labeled to ensure correct patient details.

Wash and dry hands thoroughly.

To reduce the risk of cross contamination of microorganisms.

Flush away excess proxymetacaine and fluorescein following eye examination with normal saline eye drops.

Presence of fluorescein will prevent diagnosis from conjunctival scrape.

Remove swab wand and wipe gently but firmly in inferior fornix rolling the swab to cover all surfaces.

To ensure adequate cells collected for examination by microbiologist.

Insert swab into transport container and snap off excess swab handle.
Cells will be transported in correct medium to laboratory.

Inform patient that any abnormality will be detected and the department will contact them if treatment is necessary or needs to be altered.
To keep patient informed of any changes in treatment if necessary.

Send swab in transport container with request form in a resealable plastic bag and transport to lab according to local policy.
Cells reach laboratory in timely fashion.

Document procedure according to NMC (2010) record keeping guidelines.
To ensure accurate recording in patient's notes.

Dispose of non-reusable equipment and waste into a yellow waste bin according to Trust infection control guidelines.
To comply with policies and procedures of the organisation.

Outcomes

The patient will:

understand and be able to cooperate with the investigation

be comfortable and able to maintain position during the procedure

not be exposed to the risk of cross infection

not have to repeat procedure due to unusable specimen

have correct patient details on the specimen

have sufficient cells obtained for assessment

have specimen reach laboratory in optimum condition for identification of microorganisms

not be exposed to unnecessary anxiety

have accurate record of investigation in the patient's case notes.

Viral Swab

Procedure as above but using viral swabs that are usually stored in the refrigerator – check with local policy and procedures.

Outcome

The patient will:

have correct swab used to identify viral infections.

CHLAMYDIA CONJUNCTIVAL SWAB

Standard Statement

Each patient requiring a conjunctival scrape to test for chlamydia will be fully informed of the procedure and expectation post-procedure.

Structure

The following resources are required:
- Adequate knowledge and skill to take a chlamydial swab (learner to be supervised by competent practitioner)
- Patient's medical records
- Box of tissues
- Sterile saline for irrigation
- Chlamydia swab for scrape.
- Good lighting
- Access to facilities for hand washing.

Process

The HCP should complete the following steps:

Introduce yourself to the patient, check the identity of the patient and explain the procedure including likely timeline for results.

To ensure the patient is correctly identified against the medical records and promote the patient's understanding in order to gain cooperation, obtain consent and allay anxiety.

Ensure patient is positioned comfortably reclined with head well supported.

To promote comfort and reduce head movement during procedure.

Open and label chlamydia swab from packet.

Equipment prepared and labelled to ensure correct patient details.

Wash and dry hands thoroughly.

To reduce the risk of cross contamination of microorganisms.

Flush away excess proxymetacaine and fluorescein following eye examination with normal saline eye drops.

Presence of fluorescein will prevent diagnosis from conjunctival scrape.

Ask patient to look downwards and gently evert upper eyelid.

Specimen to be taken from upper palpebral conjunctiva which has few nerve endings therefore less painful.

Using chlamydial eye swab, scrape firmly from side to side over the sub-tarsal plate until the conjunctiva blanches.

Conjunctiva will blanch when sufficient cells have been removed for diagnosis.

Insert chlamydial swab into transport container and snap off excess swab handle.

Cells will be transported in correct medium to labs.

Inform patient that tears may be blood stained for a short time.
Patient will not be alarmed by blood stained tears.

Wash and dry hands thoroughly
To reduce the risk of cross contamination of microorganisms.

Send swab in transport container with request form in a resealable plastic bag and transport to the lab according to local policy.
Cells reach lab in correct transport medium.

Document procedure according to NMC (2010) record keeping guidelines.
To ensure accurate recording in patient's notes.

Dispose of non-reusable equipment and waste into a yellow waste bin according to Trust infection control guidelines.
To comply with policies and procedures of the organization.

Outcomes

The patient will:

- understand and be able to cooperate with the investigation
- be comfortable and able to maintain position during the procedure
- not be exposed to the risk of cross infection
- have an appropriate, correctly labelled swab taken and sent for analysis
- not be exposed to unnecessary anxiety
- have accurate record of investigation in the patient's case notes.

LID TAPING FOR ENTROPION

Standard Statement

All patients with entropion will have their lower lid taped safely and effectively to prevent irritation and corneal damage. All patients will feel more comfortable, happy, and able to perform procedure themselves.

Structure

The following resources are required:
- Adequate knowledge and skill to perform and teach patient lid taping (learner to be supervised by competent practitioner)
- Transpore/Micropore tape.
- Scissors
- Mirror for patient
- Good lighting
- Tissues
- Patient medical records.

Process

The HCP should complete the following steps:

Introduce yourself to the patient, check the identity of the patient and explain the procedure to the patient including self care at home, emphasising that continued application will be necessary to prevent corneal damage until the date of minor surgery

To ensure the patient is correctly identified against the medical records and promote the patient's understanding in order to gain cooperation, obtain consent and allay anxiety.

Position the patient comfortably in a chair. Offer the patient a mirror as a teaching aid while carrying out the application of the tape.

To provide comfort while teaching the patient the method of taping lower lid.

Wash and dry hands thoroughly

To reduce risk of cross contamination with microorganisms.

Evert the patient's lower lid to the normal anatomical position.

To prevent lashes rubbing against cornea, causing irritation and infection that may result in damage to corneal surface.

Apply a piece of tape either Transpore or Micropore (if the skin is very delicate) about 4 cm long to the skin about 5 mm away from the lid margin. Ensure tape has been folded over at the end farthest from the lid margin to facilitate removal.

To correct entropion.

Ask the patient to close eyelids.

To ensure that the tape corrects the entropion but also allows good lid closure preventing exposure keratitis.

Encourage patient to practise the procedure under your supervision. A relative or friend may be taught if patient finds the technique difficult.

To ensure that the patient or relative is confident to carry out his/her treatment correctly.

Ensure that the patient has a supply of tape or is able to obtain it. Reinforce that this must continue until minor operation date. Advise the patient to contact the hospital should any related problems arise before this time.

To ensure follow-up and treatment of condition.

Document procedure according to NMC (2010) record keeping guidelines.

To ensure accurate recording in patient's notes.

Outcomes

The patient will:

understand and consent to procedure

not be exposed to risk of cross infection

have lid positioned to prevent damage to corneal surface

be discharged from hospital with all information needed to selfcare at home.

EPILATION OF INGROWING EYELASHES

Standard Statement

All patients will have their ingrown eyelashes (trichiasis) removed safely and effectively to prevent irritation and corneal damage.
All patients will give consent and feel more comfortable following the procedure.

Structure

The following resources are required:

- Adequate knowledge and skill to epilate ingrowing eyelashes
  (learner to be supervised by competent practitioner)
- Slit lamp microscope
- Sterile single use epilation forceps or sterile reusable forceps
- Sterile gauze pack
- Proxymetacaine/fluorescein single use eye drops or similar local anaesthetic drops according to local policy
- Tissues
- Patient's medical records.

Process

The HCP should complete the following steps:

Introduce yourself to the patient, check the identity of the patient and explain the procedure.

To ensure the patient is correctly identified against the medical records and promote the patient's understanding in order to gain cooperation, obtain consent and allay anxiety.

Position the patient comfortably at the slit lamp.

To provide comfort and gain cooperation and obtain good view of lashes.

Ensure adequate lighting if using magnifying glasses.

To obtain good view of ingrown lashes.

Wash and dry hands thoroughly.

To reduce risk of cross infection.

For epilation of lower lid lashes:

Gently hold lower lid down and ask patient to look upwards.

To prevent damage to cornea during procedure.

Using epilation forceps, hold lash close to base and give a sharp pull along axis until removed. Wipe forceps with sterile gauze to remove lash. Repeat process as necessary until all lashes removed.

To prevent breaking lash during removal and ensure complete removal of lash.

For removal of upper lid lashes:

Follow procedure for lower lid BUT with patient gazing downwards.
To prevent damage to cornea during procedure.

Re-examine the lashes using slit lamp or magnifying glasses explaining process to patient.
To ensure all ingrown lashes are removed and patient understands need to check for corneal damage.

Instil one drop of G. proxymetacaine/fluorescein in accordance with Patient Group Directions (PGD), or similar local anaesthetic eye drops as per local policy.
To obtain view of any corneal damage caused by ingrown lashes.

Examine patient's cornea using slit lamp and blue light or blue light on pen torch with magnifying glasses.
To identify corneal damage.

If corneal abrasion identified continue to treat patient following nurse protocols or refer to doctor in A&E.
To ensure appropriate treatment regime is followed.

Discharge patient home with appropriate information and requesting specialist review in outpatient clinic via GP referral. (Ask doctor to request referral from GP if necessary as per local protocol to ensure appropriate funds follow the patient in today's NHS.)
To ensure patient is aware of tendency to recur and the likely need for further specialist treatment if required.

Document procedure according to NMC (2010) record keeping guidelines.
To ensure accurate record in patient's medical notes.

Dispose of non-reusable equipment and waste into a yellow waste bin according to Trust infection control guidelines. Send reusable equipment to central sterilisation unit.
To comply with policies and procedures of the organisation.

Outcomes

The patient will:
understand and consent to procedure

be comfortable and able to maintain position during the procedure

have all troublesome lashes located clearly

not be exposed to risk of cross infection

have lashes removed safely and effectively

have any discomfort reduced and corneal damage effectively identified

have corneal damage identified accurately and treatment given appropriately

have sufficient knowledge about condition to be discharged safely

have accurate record of treatment in medical notes.

REMOVAL OF SUBTARSAL FOREIGN BODY (FB)

Standard Statement

All patients will be examined appropriately and have any subtarsal FB removed from superior palpebral conjunctiva.

Structure

The following resources are required:
- Adequate knowledge and skill to remove a subtarsal foreign body (learner to be supervised by competent practitioner)
- Access to hand washing facilities
- Sterile cotton buds
- Slit lamp
- G. Fluorescein and Proxymetacaine single use drops.

Process

The HCP should complete the following steps:

Introduce yourself to the patient, check the identity of the patient and explain the procedure.
To ensure the patient is correctly identified against the medical records and promote the patient's understanding in order to gain cooperation, obtain consent and allay anxiety.

Position the patient comfortably at the slit lamp.
To provide comfort, gain cooperation and obtain good view of subtarsal palpebral conjunctiva.

Wash and dry hands thoroughly.
To reduce the risk of cross contamination of microorganisms.

Evert superior eyelid to expose palpebral conjunctiva using slit lamp (when competent).
To closely examine subtarsal plate for FB.

Using a sterile cotton bud, remove FB and check palpebral conjunctiva for surface damage.
To ensure FB completely removed.

Instil one drop of G. Fluorescein and Proxymetacaine complying with appropriate PGD if competent to do so, examine corneal surface for abrasion caused by FB.
To eliminate risk of infection from undetected damage to corneal surface.

If abrasion identified, give appropriate antibiotic therapy according to PGD if competent to do so or discuss with doctor in casualty.
To prevent infection.

Document procedure according to NMC (2010) record keeping guidelines.
To ensure accurate recording in patient's notes.

Outcomes

The patient will:

understand the procedure

be able to cooperate during the procedure

not be exposed to the risk of cross infection

have palpebral conjunctiva examined completely and safely

not develop an infection following removal of FB

have accurate documentation in records to inform others.

Slit Lamp and Tonometry

Slit Lamp and Tonometry – a guide for the new ophthalmic nurse

Slit Lamp

The new nurse working in an ophthalmic area will learn many new skills as outlined within the Standard's Handbook but using a slit lamp is often the most worrying skill at first.

History

The slit lamp was created using both technical and ophthalmic expertise to create an instrument combining advanced engineering and practical experience to generate the instrument we use today. Binocular magnification, such as sphere loupe, was available prior to the end of the 19th century, invented by Edmund Hartnack in 1880. Carl Zeiss Meditec have been involved in the development of the slit lamp ever since Abbe, Zeiss and Kohler developed methods of ocular magnification which led to the development of instruments like the slit lamp (Carl Zeiss Meditec, 2001).

Dr. Gullstrand created the Gullstrand ophthalmoscope in 1911, which was manufactured by Zeiss (Carl Zeiss Meditec 2001). This was the first instrument which facilitated binocular examination of the eye using a telescopic lens connected to a vertically adjustable column moving freely on a solid base. Continued refinement and re-design occurred for the next two decades, and in 1933 Goldmann and Haag-Streit began to develop the instrument we know today. Horizontal and vertical adjustment was introduced as well as connecting the coordinated swivel motion to the cross slide facilitating examination of the anterior segment. The joystick was introduced in 1938 by Haag-Streit. This forms the basis of the slit lamp instrument that we use in ophthalmic practice today.

Effective use of the slit lamp: Shaw (2006) explains that the slit lamp enables the practitioner to use a narrow slit beam of powerful projected light producing a magnified image, facilitating examination of the eye. The ophthalmic nurse must be familiar with the slit lamp and its controls to identify the minute details that are unattainable using monocular instruments such as the direct ophthalmoscope. Madge (2006) provides useful information on the technical aspects of the slit lamp which is then supported by further detail surrounding examination using a slit lamp.

This technical aspect of the instrument is often the starting point for the nurse who wants to develop slit lamp skills. It is useful to explore the lamp itself, looking at the different components of the instrument. For example: finding out how to turn it on, checking the eyepieces are in place adjusted to the individual's personal refraction, parting the eyepieces to obtain an image from each eye then correctly aligning the eyepieces to acquire a clear binocular image and ensuring the instrument is fully mobile, unlocking the appropriate locking mechanisms.

Shaw (2006) likens using a slit lamp to driving a car. It takes practice, practice and more practice to become competent and requires support from an expert practitioner. It is often advisable to undergo a slit lamp examination to understand what it is like to be the patient. The nurse can then, under supervision, begin to use the instrument to examine the anterior segment probably starting with a willing volunteer as advised by Shaw (2006) before proceeding with 'real' patients.

Tonometry

A tonometer is an instrument that measures tension or pressure and the ophthalmic nurse will be expected to enhance their skills by measuring the intraocular pressure (IOP) of patients using a Goldmann applanation tonometer. Intraocular pressure or tension of the eye is created by the secretion, flow and drainage of aqueous humour.

History

Tension in the eye has been documented as early as the 10th century and palpation of eye tension is documented as early as 1622 (Conjoint RANZCO/RVEEH museum, 2005). We can assume that this palpation would identify patients with acute closed angle glaucoma as this causes hardening of the globe. Guthrie, an English physician, first called this hardening of the eye 'glaucoma' in 1823. Von Graefe developed the first measurement instrument in 1863. In 1885 Maklakov invented an instrument which was coated with special dye which then allowed the corneal surface to be touched using a suspension wire. The dyed end of the tonometer was then placed on special paper and the diameter of the circle produced was measured to match intraocular pressure.

Hjalmar Schiotz invented his applanation tonometer in 1905 which was further refined in 1924, the Schiotz X tonometer. With patients lying supine, this device took IOP readings by using weights to flatten or indent the cornea. Luckily, cocaine drops were available for this procedure to be carried out.

The Goldmann applanation tonometer invented in 1954 is deemed the gold standard for measuring intraocular pressure (NICE CG85, 2009).

Effective applanation tonometry: The new ophthalmic nurse will learn to use the Goldmann applanation tonometer which gives an indirect measurement using the Imbert-Flick principle (Sidebottom, 2006; Marsden, 2007). The accuracy of this measurement relies heavily on an accurately calibrated Goldmann tonometer which should be carried out before each clinic as best practice or weekly as a minimum standard (Lee, 2006). There will be occasions when Goldmann applanation tonometry cannot be performed although it is gold standard. The nurse should be familiar with Perkins tonometry (a hand-held applanation tonometer based on Goldmann principles, useful in children and anaesthetised patients). It may be suitable to use a Tono-pen® in some situations although this would not be recommended for patients with glaucoma as it is less accurate in extremes of intraocular pressure. Sidebottom (2006) and Lee (2006) both provide step-by-step guides to tonometry which may provide useful secondary information.

Pcpose (2010) highlights the limitations of Goldmann applanation tonometry due to the assumption that all corneas are uniform in thickness and rigidity. This has been shown to be inaccurate by the Ocular Hypertension Treatment study (Gordon *et al.*, 2002). This has led to the introduction of pachymetry measurements (central corneal thickness) into most ophthalmic outpatient areas as thinner than average central corneal thickness can lead to false low readings. NICE (2009) have included pachymetry as one of the investigations to be performed when assessing the patient's risk of developing open angle glaucoma. This is an investigation in which the ophthalmic nurse can develop competence and assist the clinicians in patient flow throughout the clinic.

Tonometers are calibrated to measure IOP in millimeters of mercury (mmHg) and calibration should be performed at least once a week or before every glaucoma clinic.

SLIT LAMP EXAMINATION

Standard Statement

All patients requiring nurse-led slit lamp eye examination will experience this as a professional and comfortable experience.

Structure

The following resources are required:
- Adequate knowledge and skill to clinically examine the patient using a slit lamp (learner to be supervised by competent practitioner)
- Working slit lamp complete with chin rest papers.
- Patient records
- Hard surface spray to clean lamp
- Access to hand washing facilities
- Tissues
- G. fluorescein/proxymetacaine used with prescribing rights.
- Lights dimmed to obtain best results.

Process

The HCP should complete the following steps:

Introduce yourself to the patient, check the identity of the patient and explain the procedure.
To ensure the patient is correctly identified against the medical records and promote the patient's understanding in order to gain cooperation, obtain consent and allay anxiety.

Wash and dry hands thoroughly and ensure head rest disinfected and clean chin rest paper in place.
To reduce risk of cross infection.

Position the patient comfortably on the slit lamp in a dimly lit room. Adjust the height of the table for comfort of patient and examiner. Ask patient to place chin on rest with forehead against head rest and adjust height of rest so that outer canthus is in line with demarcation line on upright support.
To provide comfort and gain cooperation and obtain good view of ocular structures.

Set up the slit lamp to suit the individual needs of the nurse when using for the first time:
- Eyepieces of bi-microscope adjusted to appropriate spectacle strength or to zero, as required and positioned for stereoscopic vision.
- Adjust the eyepieces for a clear image – focus on patient's closed eyelashes and adjust strength of refraction required.
- Adjust pupil distance until you obtain binocular view – try looking through one eyepiece at a time to ensure you have an image. If there is no image or only blackness seen adjust the eyepiece until image is obtained.
- Use one hand to operate joystick up, down, backwards and forwards.

- Use the other hand to adjust slit controls, vary angle of lamp and manipulate eyelids.

Move the illumination arm to produce a slit beam of light on the corneal surface.

To ensure focus is clear.

Light intensity switched to 5v and full beam used to systematically examine right eye structures:
- lids
- lashes
- conjunctiva
- cornea
- anterior chamber
- pupil
- lens.

Different beams and illumination angles are used when examining different structures.

- **Broad beam:** Microscope straight ahead, illumination arm 30 degrees. Set magnification at low 10x, slit wide, height 8–9 mm to examine the lids, lashes and conjunctiva. Remember to examine the superior palpebral and bulbar conjunctiva.
- **Parallel piped beam:** Microscope straight in front of patient, decrease width of beam 1–3mm, illumination arm approx. 30–45 degrees, patient looking straight ahead, remember to swing arm when scanning across structures once corneal apex achieved. This allows you to examine the corneal structures from epithelium through stroma to endothelium. You will also be able to examine the iris and the anterior surface of the lens by slowly moving your microscope forward slightly so beam is directed on to these structures.
- **Optic section:** Microscope directly in front of patient, illumination arm at 45 to 60 degrees, slit width almost closed (0.5–1mm wide by 7–9mm high), low magnification. If you position this beam within 1mm of limbus you will be able to estimate angle depth (Van Herrick estimation).
- **Conical beam:** Reduce beam to small, circular, short and narrow. Illumination arm 45–60 degrees temporally and direct across pupil, bright illumination and high magnification. Concentrate on dark area between cornea and lens to examine the anterior chamber (often the presence of cells in the aqueous looks like dust in a cinema beam (Madge 2006c)).

Van Herrick estimation – optic section near limbus with illumination arm at 60 degree, microscope directly in front of patient, look at temporal and nasal angles – compare thickness of cornea with dark section seen between front of iris and back of cornea.

Grades: 4 wide open – dark shadow equal or greater than corneal thickness

3 moderately open – ¼ to ½ corneal thickness

2 moderately narrow – closure possible – ¼ corneal thickness

1 extremely narrow – less than ¼ corneal thickness

0 – very narrow slit or no AC at all – (very rare).

To ensure all anterior segment structures are examined appropriately.

Examine both eyes systematically.

To ensure both eyes examined.

Wash hands thoroughly after the examination has concluded.

To reduce risk of cross infection.

Document procedure according to NMC (2010) record keeping guidelines.

To ensure accurate record in patient's medical notes.

Dispose of non-reusable equipment and waste into a yellow waste bin according to Trust infection control guidelines and clean slit lamp with disinfectant.

To comply with policies and procedures of the organization.

Outcomes

The patient will:

understand process and give informed consent

not be at risk of cross infection

be able to cooperate with procedure

have all structures examined systematically and thoroughly

have accurate records to inform others

have all equipment disposed of safely.

Helpful Hints

What can be easily checked when the slit lamp won't work.

1. Check the bulb

Figure 9

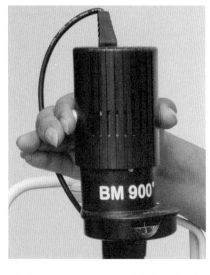

a. Loosen the screws on the side of the bulb housing.

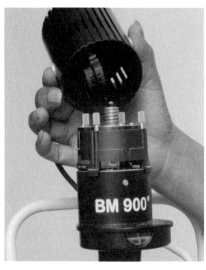

b. Lift the top of the bulb housing off carefully maintaining all electrical connections.

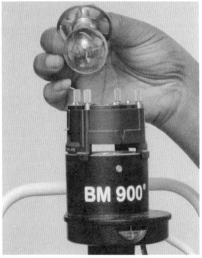

c. Check to ensure bulb is not too hot to handle and remove.

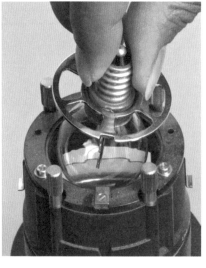

d. Examine to ensure bulb is blown and not just misaligned with contact points.

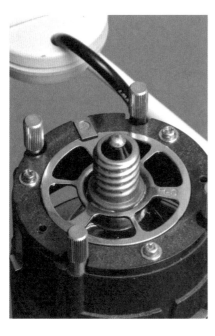

e. Replace blown bulb ensuring notch is appropriately lined up.

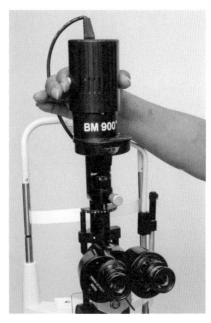

f. Reconnect the bulb housing and check beam now available.

These refer to changing the bulb on BM900 slit lamp with a similar process for the other slit lamps but these may have a slightly different locking mechanism

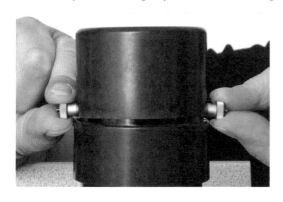

g. Alternative light bulb housing release/locking mechanism

2. Check electrical attachment still in place. (Electrical leads for some slit lamps are housed in the platform at ground level.)

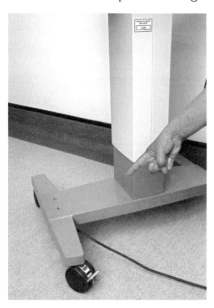

3. Ensure when you are moving the slit lamp around the departmentt that all locks are applied firmly to safeguard the slit lamp biomicroscope.

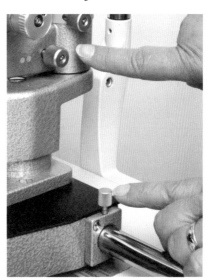

GOLDMANN APPLANATION TONOMETRY

Standard Statement

All patients requiring intraocular pressure (IOP) measurement will have it measured by Goldman applanation tonometry. This is the most commonly used accurate method of IOP measurement and is the gold standard for IOP (NICE 2009).

Structure

The following resources are required:

- Adequate knowledge and skill to perform Goldmann applanation tonometry (learner to be supervised by competent practitioner)
- Slit lamp
- Goldman applanation tonometer which has been calibrated (or personally calibrate before use – see appropriate standard) with prism either reusable or disposable as per local policy
- G. proxymetacaine and fluorescein as per PGD
- Tissues
- Sodium hypochlorite solution 10% if reusable prism is used as per local policy
- Patient case notes
- Access to hand washing facilities.

Process

The HCP should complete the following steps:

Introduce yourself to the patient, check the identity of the patient and explain the procedure.
To ensure the patient is correctly identified against the medical records and promote the patient's understanding in order to gain cooperation, obtain consent and allay anxiety.

Position the patient comfortably, ensuring privacy.
To promote cooperation and confidentiality.

Wash and dry hands thoroughly and ensure head rest disinfected and clean chin rest paper in place.
To reduce risk of cross infection.

Position the patient comfortably at the slit lamp in a dimly lit room. Adjust the height of the table for comfort of patient and examiner. Ask patient to place chin on rest with forehead against head rest and adjust height of rest so that outer canthus is in line with demarcation line on upright support.
To provide comfort and gain cooperation and obtain good view of ocular structures.

Ensure that the prism has been sterilised in sodium hypochlorite solution 10% for ten minutes or use disposable prism as per local policy.
To prevent cross infection.

Rinse prism in sterile water and wipe if a reusable prism is used or use a disposable prism. Place securely on tonometer head so that 0–180 degrees are aligned with white mark on the side.
Half circles are correctly aligned for accurate IOP reading.

Mount the tonometer on the mounting plate and turn the illuminating arm sideways to an angle of 60° and turn to blue filter. Open slit beam to widest setting, brightest light and highest voltage.
Prism illuminated correctly.

Set tonometer between numbers 1 and 2.
Normal IOP is between 10 and 21mmHg so minimal movement of calibration dial ensures quick procedure.

Instil one drop proxymetacaine/fluorescein as per Patient Group Direction or alternative prescribing method as per local policy.
Mires will be illuminated appropriately.

Re-check patient's comfort and position yourself comfortably.
Sudden movement during procedure may cause corneal epithelial damage.

Ask patient to open eyes wide or assist by retracting lids with your fingers (this may cause an involuntary squeeze and alter IOP reading).
Lids do not interfere with IOP reading. Note: Ensure fingers are not touching globe, rest fingers on orbital bones if possible otherwise compression on globe can cause raised IOP readings.

Instruct patient to look straight ahead and advance slit lamp forward until bright blue hue is seen on cornea just before touching apex (approx. 1–3 mm in front of cornea) – best seen with naked eye then move behind eye pieces.
To ensure correct position and reduce potential to cause corneal damage with prism.

Two blue/whitish half circles seen thorough eyepieces, adjacent to each other. Then gently bring prism in contact with cornea with the joystick. Yellow mires should be visible looking through left eyepiece and correctly centred horizontally and vertically.
To ensure mires are correctly placed on cornea.

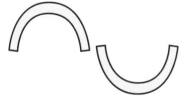

The mires should be approx. 1/10 the diameter of the semicircles.
Too much fluorescein = false high IOP – remove prism from cornea and wipe eye with tissues to remove excess fluorescein.
Too little fluorescein = false low IOP – add more proxymetacaine and fluorescein and recheck thickness of mires as above.

Turn the pressure dial until mires overlap each other as below. Read the pressure dial: 1 = 10, 2 = 20 and so on. Between 1 and 2 there are equal marks to divide the measurement into equal 2mmHg divisions. Repeat for fellow eye.
Mires appear as below when dial turned and correct IOP achieved for both eyes.

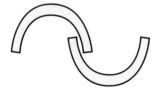

Remove prism from cornea and ask patient to sit back and relax.

To ensure patient comfort whilst recording findings in patient records.

Document procedure according to NMC (2010) record keeping guidelines including time of tonometry.

To ensure accurate record in patient's medical notes and ability to monitor IOP in relation to normal diurnal curve (higher in the morning).

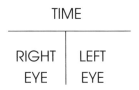

TIME

| RIGHT EYE | LEFT EYE |

Dispose of non-reusable equipment and waste into a yellow waste bin according to Trust infection control guidelines and clean slit lamp with disinfectant.

To comply with policies and procedures of the organisation.

Outcomes

The patient will:

understand process and give informed consent

not be at risk of cross infection

be comfortable and able to cooperate

not be at risk of chemical burn from sodium hypochlorite

have sufficient local anaesthetic and dye to carry out IOP test correctly

have accurate IOP reading taken

have IOP reading accurately documented in records to inform others

have all non-reusable equipment disposed of safely.

APPLANATION TONOMETRY USING A PERKINS TONOMETER

Standard Statement

All patients requiring intraocular pressure (IOP) measurement will have it measured by the handheld Perkins applanation tonometer if unable to perform Goldmann Applanation Tonometry.

Structure

The following resources are required:

- Adequate knowledge and skill to perform Perkins applanation tonometry (learner to be supervised by competent practitioner)
- Perkins applanation tonometer with prism either reusable or disposable as per local policy
- G. proxymetacaine and fluorescein as per PGD
- Tissues
- Sodium hypochlorite solution 10% if reusable prism is used as per local policy
- Patient case notes
- Access to hand washing facilities.

Process

The HCP should complete the following steps:

Introduce yourself to the patient, check the identity of the patient and explain the procedure including risk of corneal abrasion with contact tonometry.
To ensure the patient is correctly identified against the medical records and promote the patient's understanding in order to gain cooperation, obtain consent and allay anxiety.

Position the patient comfortably, ensuring privacy.
To promote cooperation and confidentiality.

Wash and dry hands thoroughly.
To reduce risk of cross infection.

Position the patient comfortably – this can be supine or sitting upright.
To provide comfort and gain cooperation and obtain good view of globe.

Ensure that the prism has been sterilised in sodium hypochlorite solution 10% for ten minutes or use disposable prism as per local policy.
To prevent cross infection.

Rinse prism in sterile water and wipe if a reusable prism is used or use a disposable prism and place securely on tonometer head so that 0–180 degrees are aligned with white mark on the side of the prism mount.

Half circles are correctly aligned for accurate IOP reading.

Move the dial on the side of the Perkins tonometer to turn on light source checking that semi-circles are illuminated before placing on to the cornea.
To ensure tonometer is ready for use preventing unnecessary repetitive corneal contact.

Instil one drop proxymetacaine/fluorescein as per patient group direction or alternative prescribing method as per local policy.
Mires will be illuminated appropriately.

Re-check patient's comfort and position yourself comfortably to the patient's side that corresponds with the eye to be examined.
Sudden movement during procedure may cause corneal epithelial damage.

Place the headrest of the Perkins tonometer on to the forehead of the patient holding it firmly with two fingers of your spare hand.
To ensure tonometer is balanced securely during use.

Ask patient to open eyes wide and to stare/focus in the distance slightly above eye level. You may assist by retracting lids with the thumb of your spare hand.
Lids do not interfere with IOP reading. Note: Ensure fingers are not touching globe, rest fingers on orbital bones if possible otherwise compression on globe can cause raised IOP readings.

Advance forward until the Perkins tonometry prism is sitting gently on the cornea.
To ensure correct position and reduce potential to cause corneal damage with prism.

Two blue/whitish half circles seen through eyepiece, adjacent to each other. Yellow mires should be visible looking through left eyepiece and correctly centred horizontally and vertically.
To ensure mires are correctly placed on cornea.

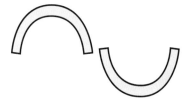

The mires should be approx. 1/10 the diameter of the semicircles.
Too much fluorescein = false high IOP – remove prism from cornea and wipe eye with tissues to remove excess fluorescein.
Too little fluorescein = false low IOP – add more proxymetacaine and fluorescein and recheck thickness of mires as above.

Turn the pressure dial on the side of the Perkins until mires overlap each other as below. Read the pressure dial: 1 = 10, 2 = 20 and so on. Between 1 and 2 there are equal marks to divide the measurement into equal 2mmHg divisions. Repeat for fellow eye.
Mires appear as below when dial turned and correct IOP achieved for both eyes.

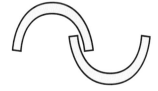

Remove prism from cornea and ask patient to sit back and relax.
To ensure patient comfort whilst recording findings in patient records.

Document procedure according to NMC (2010) record keeping guidelines including time of tonometry.
To ensure accurate record in patient's medical notes and ability to monitor IOP in relation to normal diurnal curve (higher in the morning).

TIME

RIGHT EYE	LEFT EYE

Dispose of non-reusable equipment and waste into a yellow waste bin according to Trust infection control guidelines and clean slit lamp with disinfectant.
To comply with policies and procedures of the organisation.

Outcomes

The patient will:

understand process and give informed consent

not be at risk of cross infection

be comfortable and able to cooperate

not be at risk of chemical burn from sodium hypochlorite

have sufficient local anaesthetic and dye to carry out IOP test correctly

be able to cooperate and have accurate IOP reading taken

have IOP reading accurately documented in records to inform others

have all non-reusable equipment disposed of safely.

HANDHELD TONOMETRY USING A REICHERT TONO-PEN®

Standard Statement

All patients requiring intraocular pressure (IOP) measurements will have it measured by Tono-pen, according to local policy.

Structure

The following resources are required:

- Adequate knowledge and skill to perform contact applanation tonometry (learner to be supervised by a competent practitioner).
- Reichert Tono-Pen AVIA® and Ocu-Film® tip
- Patient notes
- An office chair, not on castors that has the function of height adjustment for the patient
- Local anaesthetic drops (within expiry date) as per PGD
- Tissues
- Access to facilities for hand washing.

Process

At the beginning of a clinic, the HCP should ensure that:

1. The Reichert Tono-Pen AVIA® is visibly dust and stain free.

2. There is a supply of individual Ocu-Film® tips sealed and within expiry date.

3. For cleaning schedule, refer to Reichert Tono-Pen AVIA® manufacturer's guidelines.

Introduce yourself to the patient, check the identity of the patient and explain the procedure including the risk of corneal abrasion with contact tonometry.

To ensure the patient is correctly identified against the medical records and promote the patient's understanding in order to gain cooperation, obtain consent and allay anxiety.

Check with patient and notes for known allergies to medications and eye drops. Document any findings in patient's notes. If contact lens wearer, ask the patient to remove them before the test.

To reduce risk of adverse reactions. IOP will be inaccurate with contact lens. Promote communication between patient and the HCP.

a. Position the patient comfortably upright (ensuring privacy) using the office chair (not on castors), height adjustment if needed for the patient.

To promote cooperation and confidentiality. To provide comfort and gain cooperation and obtain good view of globe

Or

b. Position the patient comfortably in supine position.

To promote cooperation and confidentiality. To provide comfort and gain cooperation and obtain good view of globe.

Wash and dry hands thoroughly.
The HCP should follow own organisation's infection control policy on hand washing to reduce the risk of cross infection.

Instil one drop of local anaesthetic into the lower fornix without touching the eye, the lids or lashes. Offer a clean tissue. Dispose of the tissue for the patient in the nearest clinical waste bin. Offer another tissue for second eye if both eyes have IOP readings.
To prevent cross infection.

For the unregistered HCP, ensure you follow local guidelines which may include obtaining a countersignature for administration of eye drop POM. Only one drop will be held in the eye, as additional drops will spill over the lid margins. Non-contact technique for drop instillation prevents cross infection.
To ensure compliance as this procedure is uncomfortable.

Open Ocu-Film® tip (single use) and apply to transducer using a rolling action. Ensure that the Ocu-Film® tip is firmly in place. Too tight or too loose will not give accurate readings.

Calibration: this is required before using most Tono-pens.

Reichert Tono-Pen AVIA® calibration test:
Press the operating button and on the display screen 88888 will appear.
To check if machine is working accurately and ensure precision of readings.
If at this stage, these symbols do not appear, do not use. Refer to manual for troubleshooting or contact the manufacturers' helpdesk for advice.

The screen will now display = = = , followed by a bleep.

Ask the patient to gaze at a point in the distance and fix focus. Explain that they will hear a series of bleeps but to keep focus ahead. If both eyes need applanation, start with the right eye.
To keep eye still during procedure and reduce risk of corneal damage during sudden movements of the globe.

Touch the cornea gently; the machine will peep with each touch. Repeat 10 times as 10 readings are needed. After 10 readings, the Reichert Tono-Pen AVIA® will beep to signal completion. The average readings will now appear on the screen above mmHG. The statistical confidence indicator will inform the user how accurate the readings are. The HCP should aim for 95 and over. Repeat for fellow eye.

Document procedure according to NMC (2010) record keeping guidelines including time of tonometry.
To ensure accurate record in patient's medical notes and ability to monitor IOP in relation to normal diurnal curve (higher in the morning).

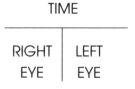

Dispose of Ocu-Film® tip according to the HCP's infection control guidelines.
To comply with policies and procedures of the organisation

This machine will automatically go to sleep mode if not used after 15 seconds. Replace in housing case.

Wash and dry hands thoroughly.

The HCP should follow own organisation's infection control policy on hand washing to reduce the risk of cross infection.

Outcomes

The patient will:

give informed consent

be able to cooperate with procedure

not be startled by beeping noises

have average of 10 readings documented in medical record.

It is good practice to keep the transducer covered with the cardboard introducer of the Ocu-Film® tip.

GOLDMANN APPLANATION TONOMETER (GAT) CALIBRATION

Standard Statement

All patients will have intraocular pressure checked with a calibrated Goldmann applanation tonometer.

Structure

The following resources are required:

- Adequate knowledge and skill to perform Goldmann applanation tonometry calibration (learner to be supervised by competent practitioner)
- Slit lamp
- Goldmann applanation tonometer platform
- Goldmann applanation tonometer prism
- Goldmann applanation tonometer calibration arm.

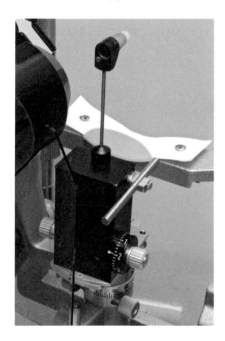

Figure 10
The calibration arm set up on
GAT platform. Remember to
move the dial to 1.

Process

The HCP should complete the following steps:

Collect your equipment.
To ensure effective time management.

Place your GAT platform on the slit lamp and insert prism. Set the GAT dial at 1.
To ensure calibration measurements are accurate.

Place the calibration arm into the side slot at the first mark from mid-point, as shown in Figure 11.
To set the arm in the correct position.

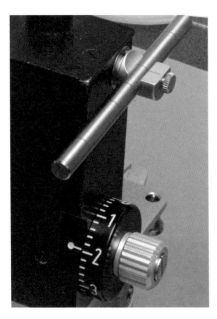

Figure 11

Slowly turn the dial towards 2 (measures 20mmHg). When the dial reaches 2, the prism should gently rock forward.

This indicates an accurate measurement at 20mmHg – turn the dial too fast and the reading will be assumed inaccurate as rock motion will happen after the 2. Measurements either one mark below or above are inaccurate.

Move the calibration arm to the second mark from mid point (at end of arm) as shown in figure 12.

To set the calibration arm to the point that measures 60mmHg.

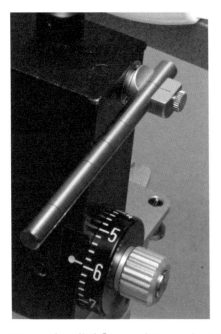

Figure 12

Move the dial forward towards 6 (measures 60mmHg). Again move dial slowly when approaching 6. Prism should rock forwards.

This indicates an accurate measurement at 60 mmHg – turn the dial too fast and the reading will be assumed inaccurate as rock motion will happen after the 6. Measurements either one mark below or above are inaccurate.

Note: if a tonometer is out of calibration you may find that there is a greater error at 6 than at 2. Hence reason to check both measurements.

Return calibration arm to storage.

Calibration should occur before every glaucoma clinic and once a week as standard.

Outcome

The patient will:

have an accurate intraocular pressure measured with a calibrated Goldmann applanation tonometer.

PACHYMETRY USING A POCKET II PACHYMETER

Standard Statement

Each patient will have central corneal thickness recorded accurately to enable IOP lowering treatment adjustments if required.

Structure

The following resources are required:

- Adequate knowledge and skill to perform pachymetry readings using a Pocket II Pachymeter (learner to be supervised by competent practitioner)
- Working Pocket II pachymeter (unnecessary to calibrate this piece of equipment as delivered calibrated. See manufacturer's manual p 37)
- Knowledge of the link between central corneal thickness (CCT) and IOP readings.
- Knowledge of the procedure
- 0.5% solution of sodium hypochlorite to disinfect probe every time this is used (see manufacturer's handbook)
- G. proxymetacaine eye drops
- Tissues
- Handwashing facilities.

Process

The HCP should complete the following steps:

Introduce yourself to the patient, check the identity of the patient and explain the procedure including risk of corneal abrasion with contact pachymetry.

To ensure the patient is correctly identified against the medical records and promote the patient's understanding in order to gain cooperation, obtain consent and allay anxiety.

Position the patient comfortably in the examination chair.

To promote cooperation and confidentiality.

Wash and dry hands thoroughly and ensure head rest disinfected and clean chin rest paper in place.

To reduce risk of cross infection.

Instil one drop of G. proxymetacaine (or alternative local anaesthetic according to local policy) into both eyes to anaesthetise the cornea. Warn the patient not to rub the eye for at least 15 minutes. If overspill needs to be removed, dab the eye with a clean tissue.

To prevent patient pain when probe touches cornea which may cause slight epithelial damage and to prevent further damage being caused by patient who may inadvertently cause a large abrasion if rubbing an anaesthetised cornea.

Whilst the drops begin to work, turn the machine on and erase any previous values using OK button.

To ensure patient values only are used by machine to average CCT.

Ask the patient to gaze at a point in the distance and fix focus. Explain that they will hear a serious of bleeps but to keep focus ahead.

To keep eye still during procedure and reduce risk of corneal damage during sudden movements of the globe.

Press measure button to start sequences (M1 will show on display). Hold the probe perpendicular to cornea at the central point (will only measure if within 10° of the perpendicular) until measurement taken.

To ensure accuracy in measurement at the appropriate place within the cornea.

Repeat the process by lifting the probe and quickly returning to cornea. Reposition if required or patient gaze moves.

To provide an average CCT reading for each patient.

The Pocket II pachymeter will take five readings in quick session ending with a long beep. This alerts the examiner that the procedure has been completed. You should review your readings as they are produced to ensure similar readings achieved.

'Bad measure' will be displayed if a measurement cannot be achieved within 45 seconds.

Document your findings in the patient record according to the NMC (2010). Pachymetry readings are displayed in microns (e.g. 566μ).

To inform other healthcare professionals of CCT values.

Outcomes

The patient will:

give informed consent

be able to cooperate with procedure

not be startled by beeping noises

have average of five readings documented in medical record.

Helpful Hints

The pachymeter works on ultrasound so if continual 'bad measure' shown, ask your patient to blink as corneal surface may have dried. Give ocular lubricant as tear film may be deficient, as necessary.

Ensure probe is perpendicular as 'bad measure' will show continually if inaccurately placed on to corneal surface.

May use four corners and centre to provide readings dependent on clinician preference. Discuss this with your consultant.

All pachymeters work in a similar fashion.

If using a different piece of equipment always consult the manufacturer's manual.

Additional Standards Using Specific Equipment

Additional Standards
Using Specific Equipment

There is a plethora of equipment available in the workplace and marketplace today to assist the ophthalmologist in their everyday practice. The ophthalmic nurse may be expected to use this equipment to aid diagnosis and provide continuous monitoring for a variety of patients with a range of clinical conditions.

All equipment will have manuals to guide the healthcare professional and nearly all companies provide training to the department when purchased to ensure that the equipment is used appropriately and accurately. The ophthalmic nurse must ensure they attend training sessions either with the company representative or with another competent healthcare professional. It would not be suitable to undertake technical procedures without adequate training. However we have written these additional standards for equipment used within our own workplace and have actually used them in clinical practice. We hope that this will provide a standard to benchmark the healthcare professional's own practice and aid the competent practitioner when supporting others in developing competent practice with the equipment outlined in this chapter. Please remember that equipment is constantly being updated and newer versions of existing equipment are introduced within the workplace. Ensure that you are completely aware of and familiar with the equipment you have available within your workplace and regularly check to ensure you are familiar with any updates installed.

DIRECT OPHTHALMOSCOPY

Standard Statement

Each patient will be competently examined using a direct ophthalmoscope.

Structure

The following resources are required:

- Adequate knowledge and skill to use a direct ophthalmoscope from the patient (learner to be supervised by competent practitioner)
- Knowledge of how the ophthalmoscope works including the limitations of the equipment (even with a dilated pupil only 1/3 of the retina can be seen).
- Knowledge of the normal retinal anatomy
- Tropicamide 1 % eye drop if required or dilating eyedrop according to local policy
- Tissues if dilating eye drops used.

Process

The HCP should complete the following steps:

Ensure the direct ophthalmoscope is working correctly with bright illumination before proceeding to patient examination – you need a white light, maximum brightness and a round circle to start.
To work efficiently and effectively to reduce patient discomfort.

Introduce yourself to the patient, check the identity of the patient and explain the procedure particularly proximity issues and temporary dazzle due to bright light.
To ensure the patient is correctly identified against the medical records and promote the patient's understanding in order to gain cooperation, obtain consent and allay anxiety.

If dilated pupil required, instil dilating eye drops according to standard (see Ocular Medications).

Position the patient comfortably, ensuring privacy and accessibility from both sides of the patient.
To promote cooperation and confidentiality.

Ask the patient to remove any spectacles.
To gain a clear view without refractive interference.

Dim the lights within the room.
To avoid background glare and maximise retinal illumination

To examine the patient's right eye stand to the right side with the direct ophthalmoscope set to '0' (zero) and a small aperture.
This ensures accessibility – do not lean across the patient.

Ask the patient to focus on a distant object such as corner of room. Be precise and reiterate the need to maintain focus even if you get in the way. The gaze should be slightly away from you, i.e. looking to the left when you examine right eye, looking to the right when you examine the left eye.
To ensure correct view is obtained including optic disc and macula and to avoid accommodation miosis (looking at a near object will make pupils constrict).

Position the ophthalmoscope in front of your right eye to examine the patient's right eye at approximately 6 inches from the patient and direct the beam into the pupil.

To obtain a red reflex and guide your approach to the patient.

It is good practice to keep both eyes open when using an ophthalmoscope but this requires practice especially when using your non-dominant eye; however it is best to start with the other eye closed.

Place your other hand on the patient's forehead with your thumb holding the upper lid.

This prevents you from colliding with the patient when you approach and allows your thumb to keep the eye open. The joint of the thumb is the exact position for your forehead to end up.

Follow the red reflex until the optic disc appears – as you approach your image will become blurred so alter the refractive dial to achieve clarity of image. Turn the dial either way, if the image becomes clearer then continue, if not reverse to turn the other way.

It is vital to obtain a clear view for accurate assessment therefore adaptation for refraction needs to be carried out.

Examine the retinal structures systematically: red reflex, anterior segment including lens opacities which show up against the red reflex, optic disc, retinal vessels (often best to use red free filter which makes blood show up black) and lastly the macula by asking patient to look directly into the ophthalmoscope.

To ensure all structures are examined for abnormalities.

Document your findings within the medical record.

To ensure accurate information shared with other healthcare professionals appropriately.

Repeat the process using left side of patient and left eye to examine patient's left eye and again document findings.

To ensure complete examination is carried out and accurate records are available.

Outcomes

The patient will:

understand what is happening and be able to cooperate with the procedure

give informed consent understanding the purpose and the side effects of the procedure

remain in correct position of gaze to facilitate procedure and reduce length of examination

be examined systematically and thoroughly with abnormalities seen

have an accurate record of examination documented to inform other healthcare professionals and clinical decision making.

➲ Helpful Hints

If you do not achieve a reasonable view, you can use one drop of a dilating drop. Wait for 15 minutes then repeat. Offer patient tissues to dab away any overspill.

You may wish to dilate a patient with small pupils in the first instance.

You must obtain patient consent and warn the patient that driving is not advisable until vision has returned to normal. Near vision especially will be affected for approximately 3–4 hours.

You will not get a clear view if you remain far away from the patient. You need to be within about 5 cm of the patient. Do not be shy; the correct position is almost cheek-to-cheek. You will need to maintain this position throughout the examination.

OPTICAL COHERENCE TOMOGRAPHY USING ZEISS STRATUS OCT™

Standard Statement

All patients requiring ocular coherence tomography (OCT) will have an accurate reading provided to the medical staff for review to inform treatment options or disease progression.

Structure

The following resources are required:

- Adequate knowledge and skill to perform OCT with the Zeiss Stratus OCT™ (learner to be supervised by competent practitioner)
- Stratus OCT™ (OCT is an optical device and measures using light waves. Coherence refers to the physical characteristics of light which allow interference patterns to form. A computer program facilitates the production of a cross section image).
- Printer paper and consumables available.
- Space to carry out procedure without distraction
- Patient medical records.

Process

The HCP should complete the following steps:

Ensure your Zeiss Stratus OCT™ machine is turned on, ready to use and sit your patient in the examination chair.
To ensure effective time management.

Introduce yourself to the patient, check the identity of the patient and explain the procedure and ask the patient to blink normally during the test until asked not to blink.
To ensure the patient is correctly identified against the medical records and promote the patient's understanding in order to gain cooperation, obtain consent and allay anxiety, obtaining quality images.

Enter the patient details as prompted by the machine: name, first and last, DOB, Hospital number.
Links print-out to unique patient identity.

Choose the programme to be used. It is possible to use for glaucoma (optic disc assessment) and retinal patients (macula assessment). This is chosen from the examination protocol.
Correct analysis is carried out by the computer program.

Position the patient comfortably and reassure the patient that although the machine will come close, it will not touch their eye. Ask the patient to focus on the green fixation dot.
To improve patient cooperation with the test.

Adjust the refraction dial and align the patient eye using the joystick (aim for the lower third of the pupil).
To enable the clearest image to be obtained.

Gently guide the scan head forward focusing through the pupil until beep is heard and align image seen in the image screen onto the fundus. The scan shape is seen on the fundus (flashing line, circle or asterisk depending on scan chosen – these may appear centrally or to either side of the screen).

To ensure correct area of the fundus, i.e. macular/optic disc, is imaged.

Observe the coloured band (the OCT image) on the left hand side of the screen and use the Z offset buttons to move image up and down if needed or press Z button if no image is apparent.
Press polarise button.

To ensure highest quality image is obtained.

Press scan mode to slow scan and begin streaming.

This allows image to be produced.

Ask the patient to hold still, continue to look at the fixation dot but reassure they can continue to blink.

To ensure patient continues to cooperate and remains comfortable.

Once the pictures are good quality (scan area clear on image, image central in the screen) ask the patient to hold still and press 'freeze without flash' button.

To ensure images are captured to facilitate analysis. 'Without flash' is used to facilitate further scans if required.

Ask the patient to sit back and relax whilst analysis takes place.

To reduce patient discomfort.

Press review and the last eight sets of images will appear on the screen. Review and save the best image.

To ensure the images are saved for review by clinician if required and for future analysis against another set of images.

Return to the main menu to analyse the images by pressing the 2 people icon at the top of the screen. Analyse using program requested by clinician e.g. retinal thickness single eye, RNFL (retinal nerve fibre layer) single eye.

To ensure correct analysis takes place and facilitate accurate print out of information.

Print a copy of the information for review by clinician and storage in patient record.

To ensure patient record is up-to-date and contemporaneous to facilitate accurate diagnosis, further treatment and meet legal requirements for record keeping.

Sign and date the entry.

To act in accordance with professional guidelines for records and record keeping.

Outcomes

The patient will:

give consent to procedure

be able to cooperate without discomfort

have accurate quality images produced from the scan

have good quality images saved within the computer program for the doctor to review if required.

OPTICAL COHERENCE TOMOGRAPHY USING ZEISS CIRRUS OCT™

Standard Statement

All patients requiring ocular coherence tomography (OCT) will have an accurate reading provided to the medical staff for review to inform treatment options or disease progression.

Structure

The following resources are required:

- Adequate knowledge and skill to perform OCT with the Zeiss Cirrus OCT™ learner to be supervised by competent practitioner)
- Cirrus OCT™ (OCT is an optical device and measures using light waves. Coherence refers to the physical characteristics of light which allow interference patterns to form. A computer program facilitates the production of a cross section image)
- Printer paper and consumables available
- Space to carry out procedure without distraction
- Patient medical records.

Process

The HCP should complete the following steps:

Ensure your Zeiss Cirrus OCT™ machine is turned on, ready to use and sit your patient in the examination chair.

To ensure effective time management.

Introduce yourself to the patient, check the identity of the patient and explain the procedure and ask the patient to blink normally during the test until asked not to blink.

To ensure the patient is correctly identified against the medical records and promote the patient's understanding in order to gain cooperation, obtain consent and allay anxiety, obtaining quality images.

Enter the patient details as prompted by the OCT if this is the first time an OCT scan has been performed: name, first and last, DOB, Hospital number and press Save.

Links print out to unique patient identity. If previous scans have been performed use the Find Existing Patient screen to find your patient.

Once the patient has been found, locate and press the acquire button at the base of the screen. The acquire screen will then be displayed.

To be able to proceed to the scan.

Choose the program to be used. It may be used for glaucoma (optic disc assessment – optic disc cube) and retinal patients (macula assessment – macula cube: usually macula cube 512x128 is used but if in doubt, ask the doctor which program he/she requires). This is located at the top of the acquire screen.

Correct analysis is carried out by the computer program.

Position the patient comfortably and reassure the patient that although the machine will come close, it will not touch their eye.

To improve patient cooperation with the test.

To assess the right eye the patient should place his/her chin on the chin rest at the blue indicator line with their forehead pressed against the blue indicator line on the forehead support. The eye should be aligned with the mark at the side of the chinrest/forehead apparatus similar to the black line on the slit lamp.

To ensure the scan is taken from the correct eye. This may be unusual for the patient as they are used to placing their chin in the centre of the slit lamp chin rest and resting forehead centrally against the forehead support. You may need to guide the patient in the first instance.

The OD circle should now highlight blue at the top of the screen to indicate the right eye is being scanned.

To ensure correct eye is being scanned.

The upper left hand side of the screen facing the examiner should show the eye but the examiner can use the 'X–Y' controls to the right of this picture to move the red scan light to the pupil and use the chin rest arrows to move the chin rest back and forth. The examiner can also place the cursor on to the centre of the pupil and left click the mouse to allow the machine to centre the scan through the pupil. Warn the patient that the chin rest may move independently.

Tell the patient to focus on the centre of the green star within the machine – this is placed centrally for a macula scan and off to the left for an optic disc scan.

To obtain adequate view of the macula or optic disc. The lower left hand side of the screen or fundus view port will show a black and white picture of these areas when correctly positioned.

Check the fundus view port screen for the overlying box which indicates the location of the scan with a small green cross in the centre indicating the location of the fixation target. Click the 'Auto Focus' to ensure adequate focus then click 'Optimize', both are located to the right of the fundus view port.

To ensure optimum scan obtained.

Tell the patient to blink just before starting to capture the image then not to blink whilst image capture in progress and click 'Capture', again located to the right of the fundus view port.

To obtain scan of relevant retinal structure.

Once the scan has completed, the Review Scan screen appears automatically. Check the signal strength (upper centre of screen) which should be highlighted in green and no less than 6 but the higher values are preferred.

To assess quality of scan obtained.

If the captured scan is of good quality click Save at the bottom of this screen but if of poor quality press 'Try again'. This will then return to the Acquire screen so that a repeat scan can be performed. Repeat the process until you have obtained a scan of good quality with signal strength of 6 or above.

To ensure good quality scans are stored for analysis.

Repeat the process for the left eye by asking the patient to move their chin and forehead to the white indicator line. Note: for optic disc scans the green star will appear to the right of the screen.

To ensure quality scan obtained and stored for analysis.

When you are certain that good quality scans have been obtained click 'Finish' located at the bottom of the screen on the right hand side which returns automatically to the Find patient screen.

The patient can then relax back from the OCT.

To promote comfort whilst the analysis takes place.

Click on Today's Patient screen and click on the individual patient name. Acquire and Analyze will then be highlighted at the bottom of the screen. Click on 'Analyze'.

To ensure accurate patient scans are analysed.

Identify the scans to be used from the top of the screen, left hand side and the program to be used for analysis, right hand side.

To ensure accurate analysis takes place.

Outcomes

The patient will:

> understand the procedure and give consent
> be able to cooperate throughout the procedure
> have accurate high quality images saved for the clinician to review.

Helpful Hints

- When analysing the optic cube 200x200, the usual program is ONH + RNFL OU Analysis.
- When analysing the macula cube 512x128, the usual program is macula thickness.

Remember: you can always ask the doctor or appropriate healthcare professional which program they wish to be used and they may wish to review the scans on the OCT to access 3D visualisation and other programs available within the Zeiss Cirrus OCT™.

Click on the Print icon (top right hand corner) to access the Print screen. Once in the Print screen click Print (top left hand corner)

To ensure appropriate scans are printed and documented in the patient's medical records.

If appropriate, ask the patient to wait outside the correct clinical examination room for review by the suitable healthcare professional or doctor.

TOPOGRAPHY USING AN OCULUS PENTACAM®

Standard statement

All patients requiring corneal topography will have this measured by a competent practitioner using an Oculus Pentacam®.

(Topography is defined as the science of representing the features of particular places in detail, in this case the cornea. There are three refractive elements of the eye, axial length, lens and cornea, and the cornea has the highest refractive power. This is of vital importance when considering refractive elements of cataract surgery, as well as assessment of keratoconus.)

Structure

The following resources are required:

- Adequate knowledge and skill to perform topography
  (learner to be supervised by competent practitioner)
- Oculus Pentacam®
- Hard surface disinfectant according to local policy
- Tissues
- Patient medical records
- Private area for assessment free from distraction.

Process

The HCP should complete the following steps:

Introduce yourself to the patient, check the identity of the patient and explain the procedure.
To ensure the patient is correctly identified against the medical records and promote the patient's understanding in order to gain cooperation, obtain consent and allay anxiety.

Switch on the PC attached to the Oculus Pentacam® and then turn on the Pentacam itself.
The Pentacam will communicate with the PC to store all the measurements saved.

Clean the forehead support and table with the appropriate hard surface spray or other as local policy dictates, removing the top chin rest paper.
To reduce the risk of cross infection.

Double click on the Pentacam logo with the computer mouse to access Patient ID input screen, enter patient details and click on 'Save Data'. Confirm whether this is a new episode for a new patient or a further episode for known patient.
To ensure accurate details of individual are entered into the system for a new patient or locate previous scans stored within the system.

Position the patient comfortably at the appropriate height with medial canthus meeting the marker on the side of the chin rest/forehead apparatus ensuring privacy within the examination area.
To promote cooperation and confidentiality.

Click on 'Examination' and click 'Scan' from drop down box. Ask the patient to look directly ahead at the blue slit light with the eye to be measured.

This ensures good fixation for accurate scans to be obtained.

Using the joy stick:

- move the Pentacam until the blue light is in the middle of the selected cornea
- move the Pentacam slowly forward until the lids and cornea can be seen in the main screen.
- observing the target screen, centralise the cornea until the three straight lines become crisp and the yellow cross is centred in the target.

Central corneal area will be within the scanning range and promote accurate scans.

- instruct the patient to stare at the blue light with wide eyes and to try not to blink
- advance Pentacam slowly until the red dot on the cornea almost meets the line
- instruct the patient to take a long blink and then open their eye very wide
- Pentacam will automatically take the scan when the optimum position is achieved
- encourage the patient to keep their eyes wide open during the seconds that the scan is being taken.

To promote a good corneal scan without eyelids obstructing the cornea.

If there is difficulty getting the Pentacam to initiate the measurement due to dry-looking tear film, get the patient to blink forcibly a few times and repeat the process.

A moist cornea promotes a better quality scan.

Advise patient to sit back while scans are evaluated. Comments may be 'blink' indicating inadequate corneal surface, or the K's may be highlighted in red or yellow and will need to be repeated.

To ensure that the best possible quality scans are available.

If scans are of appropriate quality, or of the best quality obtainable due to corneal pathology click on 'Display', and click on 'Holladay'. Print Holladay Report.

These are the most common scans requested for cataract surgery. However the doctor may request further print outs of scans if necessary.

Repeat process for fellow eye if clinically indicated, e.g. in keratoconus.

Scans of both eyes are able to be evaluated.

Store in the patient's medical records.

Scans will be safely and confidentialy stored and available for further assessment by the appropriate healthcare professional.

Outcomes

The patient will:

be able to understand and cooperate with the scanning process

have accurate scans documented within their individual medical records.

Next Steps using Standards

Next Steps using Standards

Each nurse needs to keep a portfolio of development for the Nursing and Midwifery Council to be able to re-register every year (NMC, 2008). Re-registration requires the registrant (the registered nurse) to provide evidence of 35 hours of learning activity (Continuing Professional Development) in the previous three years. This handbook with its associated competency assessment suggested document would provide clear evidence of learning activities within the workplace.

We suggest the ophthalmic nurse use the standards to validate current practice thereby quality assuring the individual's practice. The nurse new to working within an ophthalmic environment will discuss their development with their line manager and find an experienced ophthalmic nurse to act as a guide or mentor. The individual and the guide should jointly decide a direction of development using the appropriate standards as the assessment criteria. It may be wise to have this initial discussion fairly quickly so that the individual nurse develops appropriately and effectively.

The non-registered nurse will also need to develop competencies for the skills they use in their clinical practice. These skills are usually developed by working alongside a registered nurse who is responsible for delegating such activities to the non-registered nurse. This delegation of procedures will obviously be discussed with the ophthalmic clinical manager following appropriate risk assessments to ensure each organisation accepts vicarious liability for each delegation. These standards and appropriate assessment strategies can be employed to provide evidence of the safe practice for the non-registered nurse.

The individual registered nurse is responsible for their own development and ensuring they are competent in the skills they need to deliver safe and effective clinical practice. The non-registered nurse may need guidance but should accept responsibility for working within the parameters of the job description unless in an agreed pathway of development.

We suggest that each procedure should be observed by the competent practitioner a minimum of 10 times before attempting assessment. All nurses regardless of grade or registration should only work within their own level of competence but should take steps to develop in accordance with local policy and guidance that are available within each employing Eye Unit.

SUGGESTED FORMAT FOR PROVIDING EVIDENCE OF DEVELOPMENT AND COMPETENCE

We suggest that this may be used to identify the relevant personnel involved in the development of the individual.

AUTHORISED SIGNATORIES

NAME	PLACE OF WORK	DESIGNATION	SIGNATURE	INITIALS

INITIAL DISCUSSION/PLAN FOR FUTURE DEVELOPMENT

INITIAL DISCUSSION
NAME OF NURSE   NAME OF GUIDE/MENTOR
Practice learning opportunities and competencies discussed
Action plan to maximise achievement of learning opportunities and competencies
Skills identified
Date identified for achieving initial competencies
Signature of nurse   Signature of mentor

CONTINUED DEVELOPMENT

Competencies Achieved
Further development identified
Strategies for achieving new competencies:
Date agreed for further development success: Nurse signature Mentor signature

EVIDENCE OF PRACTICE – Main Outpatient Area (this may be changed to the relevant area of practice, e.g. Accident & Emergency, Day Surgery unit)

DATE	SKILL	KEY LEARNING

SUGGESTED COMPETENCE ASSESSMENT DOCUMENTATION

Visual Acuity Testing

Criteria	Assessor's comments to demonstrate criteria met
Prepare individual and equipment:	**Date:**
Ensure appropriate VA testing equipment available	
Case notes of individual	
Infection control measures: Patient Personal hygiene	
Inform patient why accurate VA is required	
Patient is made comfortable	
VISUAL ACUITY TESTING	
Identifies correct test to be used for individual patient	
Prepares patient by explaining procedure	
Checks patient understands what is required during the procedure and consent is given	
Documents all information given by patient/relative accurately.	
Demonstrates competence in:	
Snellen chart	
Sheridan–Gardiner	
E cube test	
Kays Picture test	
Responds to patient throughout the procedure	
Correct documentation completed	
Escorts patient & relative to waiting area outside relevant doctor's clinic room.	
Ensures notes are given to doctor to make certain patient is seen by doctor in an efficient manner	Assessor's Signature:

History Taking

Criteria	Assessor's comments to demonstrate criteria met
Prepare individual and equipment:	**Date:**
Appropriate documentation available	
Case notes for individual patient	
Infection control measures: Personal hygiene	
Inform patient why accurate history is required	
Patient is made comfortable	
HISTORY TAKING :	
Obtains accurate information about nursing, medical and medication history efficiently and effectively using correct documentation or medical records	
Questions from patient and/or relative are answered clearly and concisely	
Documents all information given by patient/relative accurately.	
Ensures patients understand what information is required and why	
Undertakes visual acuity testing prior to instillation of dilating eye drops	
Checks for RAPD prior to instilling eye drops (see competency assessment)	
Instils dilating eye drops appropriately (see competence assessment)	
Correct documentation completed	
Escorts patient & relative to waiting area outside relevant doctor's clinic room.	
Ensures notes are given to doctor to make certain patient is seen by doctor in an efficient manner	
Correct documentation completed	
Escorts patient & relative to waiting area outside relevant doctor's clinic room.	Assessor's Signature:
Ensures notes are given to doctor to make certain patient is seen by doctor in an efficient manner	

Non-contact Biometry

Criteria	Assessor's comments to demonstrate criteria met
Prepare individual and equipment:	**Date:**
Documentation: ICP	
Equipment: IOL Master checked & calibrated Correct and adequate	
Infection control measures: Patient Equipment Personal hygiene	
Inform patient	
Confirm identity and entered accurately on IOL Master	
Get consent	
Identify eye to be operated on	
Patient is made comfortable	
NON-CONTACT BIOMETRY:	
Questions answered clearly and concisely	
Instructions given clearly & concisely	
Axial length measured and checked for both eyes	
Similar measurements or correct action taken if dissimilar	
Corneal curvature measurements performed and checked against spectacle prescription	
When there is a problem remedial action is taken	
Patient is seated comfortably away from machine when measurements obtained	
IOL calculation performed using: Correct formula Correct surgeon	
Information for IOL printed	Assessor's Signature:
Filed in patient notes	
Correct documentation completed	

Irrigation of Eye Following Chemical Injury

Criteria	Assessor's comments to demonstrate criteria met
Prepare individual and equipment:	**Date:**
Ensure all equipment required available for use.	
Casenotes of individual patient available if relevant.	
Infection control measures – hand washing.	
Inform patient why procedure is necessary.	
Patient reclined comfortably.	
IRRIGATION OF EYE FOLLOWING CHEMICAL INJURY:	
If patient attending A&E with acutely presenting chemical injury irrigate eye prior to obtaining personal details. Establish basic general health and allergies. Delay in irrigation will cause further damage.	
If not acute, obtain personal details and establish pH of the eye.	
Explain procedure to patient, establish understanding and obtain informed consent.	
Instil local anaesthesia to affected eye.	
Irrigate eyelids and eye through all extremities of gaze and though upper and lower fornices with a minimum of a litre of sterile saline.	
Wait for 10 minutes and assess pH.	
If pH 7, assess patient and pass patient though to Dr for ocular assessment.	
If pH > 7, continue irrigation until pH returns to 7.	
Dispose of clinical waste according to hospital policy.	
Dr reviews patient and prescribes treatment.	
Ensure patient understands importance of compliance with treatment and provide review appointment if necessary.	**Assessor's Signature:**
Patient informed to return for review prior to appointment if any deterioration of condition.	

As you can see the competence assessment document can be as large and detailed as you wish. The more complex the task, the more detailed the assessment document needs to be. We have only suggested ways that the individual nurse can provide evidence of their skills and competence.

BLANK TEMPLATE FOR STANDARD SETTING

Standard Statement

Write a statement that sets out what the patient should expect from the intervention or procedure.

Structure

Identify all the elements that you will need to carry out the procedure i.e. knowledge, skill, confidence, equipment. Be as specific as you can.

Process

Identify each step you will take to complete the procedure, and state why you take each step. Ensure this meets with national guidance and up-to-date evidence.

Outcome

The outcome for the standard should be expressed in terms of patient outcomes rather than practitioner outcomes.

BLANK TEMPLATE FOR ASSESSMENT

Criteria	Assessor's comments to demonstrate criteria met
Prepare individual and equipment:	Date:
NAME OF PROCEDURE:	
	Assessor's Signature:

We hope that this will be a logical starting point for all nurses/healthcare professionals to track their skills and competence. Obviously these standards and assessment documents can also be used to validate competence once in a while during the course of all our careers.

References

Carl Zeiss Meditec AG (2001) *Eye Examination with the Slit Lamp*. Available on line at: http://www.zeiss.com/8825 6DE3007B916B/0/506FBA0E8FCB598E882571D8007D4B40/$file/spaltlampen_eye_exam_en.pdf (Last accessed 23.09.11).

Colenbrander, A. (2001) *The Historical Evolution of Visual Acuity Measurement* available at: http://www.ski.org/Colenbrander/Images/HIstory_VA_Measurement.pdf [accessed 28.9.11].

Conjoint The Royal Australian and New Zealand College of Ophthalmologists/The Royal Victorian Eye and Ear Hospital (RANZCO/RVEEH) museum (2005) *The Measurement of Intraocular Pressure* available on line at: http://www.rveeh.vic.gov.au/library/Museum/Intraocular_pressure.htm (Last accessed 23.09.11).

Davies, H. (2006) 'Patient Education' in Marsden, J. (Ed.) (2006) *Ophthalmic Care,* Chichester:Whurr Publishers Ltd.

Department of Health (1998) *A First Class Service: Quality in the new NHS.* London: The Stationery Office.

Department of Health (2008) *National Patient Survey.* available at: www.dh.gov.uk/en/Publicationsandstatistics/Publications/PublicationsStatistics/DH_098859 (Last accessed 23.09.11).

Elliott, D.B. (2003) *Clinical Procedures in Primary Eye Care*. Edinburgh: Butterworth Heinemann.

Field D. 2009 Basic Ophthalmic Procedures IN Field D., Tillotson J. & MacFarlane M. 2009 *The Ophthalmic Study Guide for Nurses & Health Professionals* Keswick: M&K Publishing.

Field, D. and Tillotson J. (2008) *Eye Emergencies: A Practitioner's Guide*. Keswick: M&K Publishing.

Gordon, M.O., Beiser, J., Brandt, J.D., Heuer, D.K., Higginbotham, E.J., Johnson, C.A., Keltner, J.L., Miller, J.P., Parrish, R.K.,2nd., Wilson, M.R. and Kass, M.A. (2002) 'The Ocular Hypertension Treatment Study: baseline factors that predict the onset of primary open angle glaucoma.' *Archive of Ophthalmology* **120**: 714–720.

Kanski, J. (2007) *Clinical Ophthalmology: A Systematic Approach* 7th Edn. Edinburgh: Butterworth Heinemann.

Ledford, J.K. (1999) *The Complete Guide to Ocular History Taking*. Thorofare, NJ: Slack Publications.

Lee, A. (2006) 'The Angle and the Aqueous' in Marsden, J. (Ed.) (2006) *Ophthalmic Care*. Chichester: Whurr Publishers Ltd.

Madge, S.N. (2006a) 'A suggested scheme for refraction' in Madge, S.N., Kersey, J.P., Hawker, M.J. and Lamont, M.(Eds) (2006) *Clinical Techniques in Ophthalmology*. Edinburgh: Churchill Livingstone.

Madge, S.N. (2006b) 'Examination of the Pupils' in Madge, S.N., Kersey, J.P., Hawker, M.J. and Lamont, M. (Eds) (2006) *Clinical Techniques in Ophthalmology*. Edinburgh: Churchill Livingstone.

Madge, S.N. (2006c) 'Technical Use of the Slit Lamp' in Madge, S.N., Kersey, J.P., Hawker, M.J. and Lamont, M (Eds) (2006) *Clinical Techniques in Ophthalmology*. Edinburgh: Churchill Livingstone.

Marsden, J. (2006) 'The Care of patients presenting with acute problems' in Marsden, J. (Ed.) (2006) *Ophthalmic Care.* Chichester: Whurr Publishers Ltd.

Marsden, J. (2007) *An Evidence Base for Ophthalmic Nursing Practice.* Chichester: John Wiley & Sons Ltd.

Morell, C., Harvey, G. and Kitson, A. (1997) Practitioner Based Quality Improvement: A review of the Royal College of Nursing's dynamic standard setting system, *Quality in Healthcare* **6** (1), 29–34.

National Eye Institute (1999) *Early Treatment Diabetic Retinopathy Study (ETDRS)* available at: http://clinicaltrials.gov/ct2/show/NCT00000151 (accessed 28.9.11).

NICE (2009) *Glaucoma Diagnosis and Management of Chronic Open Angle Glaucoma and Ocular Hypertension* available on line at: http://www.nice.org.uk/nicemedia/live/12145/43839/43839.pdf (Last accessed 23.09.11).

Nursing and Midwifery Council (2008) *The Code* available at: http://www.nmc-uk.org/Nurses-and-midwives/The-code/The-code-in-full/ (accessed 21.2.11).

Nursing and Midwifery Council (2008) *The PREP Handbook* available at: http://www.nmc-uk.org/Educators/Standards-for-education/The-Prep-handbook/ (accessed 12.4.11).

Nursing and Midwifery Council (2010) *Record Keeping: Guidance for Nurses and Midwives* available at: http://www.nmc-uk.org/Documents/Guidance/ nmcGuidanceRecordKeepingGuidanceforNursesandMidwives.pdf (accessed 21.2.11).

Pepose, J. (2010) *Measuring Intraocular Pressure, Advanced Ophthalmic Care.* available at: http://www.peposevision.com/pdf/measuring-intraocular-pressure_7_2010.pdf (Last accessed 16.10.11).

Ring, L. (2010) *I want my eye nurse to be......* Audit presentation at RCN Ophthalmic Forum conference, (unpublished).

Royal College of Nursing (1990) *Quality Patient Care: the Dynamic Standard Setting System*. Harrow: Scutari.

Shaw, M. (2006) 'Examination of the Eye' in Marsden, J. (Ed) (2006) *Ophthalmic Care*. Chichester: Whurr Publishers Ltd.

Shaw, M.E., Lee, A. and Stollery, R. (2010) *Ophthalmic Nursing*, 4th Ed. Chichester: John Wiley & Sons Ltd.

Sheridan, M. and Gardiner, P. (1970) 'Sheridan-Gardiner Test for Visual Acuity'. *British Medical Journal*. available at: http://www.ncbi.nlm.nib.gov/pmc/articles/PMC1699941/pdf/brmedj02283-0062.pdf (accessed 28.9.11).

Sidebottom, R. (2006) 'Tonometry' in Madge, S.N., Kersey, J.P., Hawker, M.S. and Lamont, M (Eds) (2006) *Clinical Techniques in Ophthalmology*. Edinburgh: Churchill Livingstone/Elsevier.

Van der Wiel, H.L. and Van Gijn, J. (1986) 'The Diagnosis of Horner's Syndrome: Use and limitations of the cocaine test' *Journal of Neurological Sciences* **73** (3), 311–316.

Whittaker, L. (2006). 'Visual Impairment' in Marsden, J (Ed.) (2006) *Ophthalmic Care*. Chichester: Whurr Publishers Ltd.

Websites

History and Heritage. Available at http://www.reichert.com/history.cfm (Accessed 19/04/2011)

History of Cocaine. Available at http://www.cocamuseum.com/htm/historycocaine.htm (Accessed 19/04/2011)

Tonometers. Available at http://www.college-optometrists.org/en/knowledge-centre/museyeum/online_exhibitions/optical_instruments/tonometers.cfm (Accessed 19/04/2011)

Further reading

Fercher, A. and Roth, E. (1986) 'Ophthalmic Laser Interferometer'. *Proceedings of SPIE* **658**, 48–51.

IOL Master Online Instructions Manual v.5.
Available from http://doctor-hill.com/zeiss_iolmaster/iolmaster-manual.htm (Last accesssed 23.09.11).

Oliver, F. (2005) 'Biometry and Intraocular Lens Power Calculation.' *Current Opinion in Ophthalmology* **16** (1), 61–64.

Parker, M., Fine, H., Hoffman, R.S.,Coffman, P.G, and Brown, L.K .(2002) 'Immersion A-scan Compared with Partial Coherence Interferometry: Outcomes analysis.' *Journal of Cataract & Refractive Surgery* **28** (2): 239–242.

Royal College of Ophthalmologists (2010) 'Cataract Surgery Guidelines.' September 2010.
Available from http://www.rcophth.ac.uk (Last accessed 23.09.11)